150 Commonly Prescribed Drugs

150 Commonly Prescribed Drugs:

A guide to their uses and side effects

by
Edward R. Brace
Fellow, American Medical Writers Association

Special Consultant
Arthur Hull Hayes, Jr., M.D.
Professor of Medicine and Pharmacology
The Pennsylvania State University

Published by

World Book–Childcraft International, Inc.
A subsidiary of The Scott & Fetzer Company

Chicago London Paris Sydney Tokyo Toronto

Contents

Introduction

The purpose of this book is to present facts about 150 of the drugs most often prescribed by physicians each year in the United States. Information is given on the general class of each drug, in what dosage form the drug is available, why it is prescribed, possible side effects associated with the use of the drug, general background information you should know about the drug, and special precautions you should observe during its use.

One of the features of this book is the list of "possible" adverse reactions (side effects) that sometimes can occur in certain patients. At first reading, this list can be quite alarming. Certain drugs can produce unwanted effects in some persons. That is, if a drug is powerful enough to exert a therapeutic effect on the body or control the course of a disease, it is occasionally likely to exert other effects as well. However, it is essential to understand that adverse reactions do not occur in everyone who takes a particular drug; nor do they occur each and every time that the drug is taken. The list of side effects for each drug included in this book are only "possible" reactions encountered by some persons using the drug.

Drugs available only by a physician's prescription (ethical pharmaceuticals) are generally much more potent than those which are freely available at any drugstore without a prescription (over-the-counter or OTC drugs). There are several exceptions to this rule. For example, aspirin is an extremely effective and potent drug which does not require a prescription. Some people are extremely sensitive to aspirin and can experience serious side effects such as bleeding from the stomach. Thus, it is a mistake to think that only a drug available by a physician's prescription can cause unwanted effects. All drugs must be treated with great respect and taken exactly as the label or the physician directs.

The incidence of potentially serious adverse reactions with the safe and proper use of most prescription drugs is very low. In some cases, the possibility of a potentially serious side effect occurring may be preferable to withholding the drug, especially if the condition being treated is a direct threat to life. In other cases, this possibility is not justified because the condition being treated is relatively minor.

It is important to notify your physician at once if you experience any side effect while taking a drug he or she has prescribed for you. Your physician is the most qualified judge of what drugs you should or should not take. He or she will then decide whether to reduce the dose of the drug, or prescribe another drug to achieve the most beneficial results.

The Food and Drug Administration (FDA) has established rigid guidelines about both the relative safety and the effectiveness of prescription drugs. Before a drug can be prescribed by your physician, it must be submitted to extensive tests. This usually includes administration of the drug to various species of laboratory animals. If the drug passes all of the required tests and procedures, the manufacturer is given permission to market it under a brand name.

Once the patent for a brand name drug expires, the product is often made available under its chemical or *generic* name. Many chemically identical drugs are available under several brand names. Others are available under one or more brand names in addition to the drug's generic name. Generally speaking, if your physician prescribes a drug under its generic name it will be considerably less expensive than if the brand name of the drug is written on the prescription pad.

Most of the drugs discussed in this book are entered in alphabetical order under the most commonly prescribed brand names. A few are listed under their chemical or generic names, such as tetracycline and erythromycin, and immediately beneath them appears a list of some of the leading brand names.

Thousands of different drugs are prescribed in the United States each year, although in many cases, they tend to achieve about the same therapeutic effects within their class. This book includes twenty-six separate drug classes. Among these are: antibacterials, antihistamines and decongestants, antihypertensives (for the treatment of high blood pressure), anti-inflammatory drugs, antitussives (cough suppressants), oral contraceptives, analgesics (pain relievers), tranquilizers and antidepressants, sedatives, and anticonvulsants.

Some prescription drugs contain only a single chemical ingredient. Others contain a combination of two or more different ingredients. These "fixed-combination" drugs are prescribed if the physician believes that the combined therapeutic effects of the ingredients are just right for a particular patient.

The pharmaceutical industry has truly revolutionized modern medicine. With this revolution, various problems have emerged. Physicians, for example, must be continually informed by drug manufacturers about the proper use of new drugs; their therapeutic indications and the special precautions involved in their use. Patients and their families also have the right to know more about the drugs they take. They have the right to know what a specific drug is designed to do and what adverse effects have been reported in patients taking the drug even though serious reactions may be relatively rare. By being so informed, an individual can become a better patient.

We hope that this book will help patients and their families to become better informed about the 150 leading drugs prescribed each year in the United States.

A-Z drug list

Actifed®

Generic name
This product contains a combination of triprolidine
hydrochloride and pseudoephedrine hydrochloride.

Class of drug
Antihistamine plus a decongestant

In what form is the drug available?
Tablets and syrup

Why is the drug prescribed?
It is designed to relieve the symptoms of a.stuffy nose
or nasal congestion (swelling of the tissues that line
the nose) in conditions such as hay fever or the
common cold. The drug is also claimed to be effective
in controlling the symptoms of mild and uncomplicated
skin allergies such as itching, swelling, or hives, and
to relieve the symptoms of allergic conjunctivitis.
Thus, its major sites of action are the nose, the skin,
and the eyes.

What are some possible side effects?

The most frequently encountered side effects are drowsiness, sedation, dizziness, disturbed coordination, thickening of secretions in the lower air passages (bronchial tubes), and excessive dryness of the nose, mouth, and throat. However, some patients have experienced more serious reactions while taking Actifed. These include: a rapid beating or fluttering of the heart, extreme nervousness, blurred vision, hallucinations, and convulsions.

What should you know about the drug?

The FDA, based partly on a review of this drug by the National Academy of Sciences, states that it is "probably" effective for the treatment of symptoms of allergic rhinitis (hay fever) and related conditions. However, they also state that there is a lack of "substantial evidence of effectiveness as a fixed combination" for the prevention and treatment of symptoms of the common cold.

Are there any special precautions?

The drug should not be given to newborn or premature infants or to nursing mothers. It should not be used to treat patients with asthma or other disorders of the lower respiratory tract. And it should not be given to persons with a known adverse reaction to antihistamines.

Actifed must be used with extreme caution (if at all) in patients with a particular form of glaucoma (narrow-angle glaucoma), obstruction of the neck of the bladder, diabetes, heart disease, high blood pressure, or an overactive thyroid gland (hyperthyroidism).

Actifed-C® Expectorant

Generic name

This product contains a combination of codeine phosphate, glyceryl guaiacolate, pseudoephedrine hydrochloride, triprolidine hydrochloride, and preservatives.

Class of drug

Antitussive, expectorant, decongestant, and antihistamine

In what form is the drug available?

Syrup

Why is the drug prescribed?

This drug is designed to provide four distinct therapeutic actions: (1) suppress coughing associated with
either infections or allergies that affect the respiratory
tract; (2) reduce the thickness of secretions in the air
passages thus aiding in their removal by the cough
reflex; (3) open up air passages narrowed by congestion; (4) provide antihistaminic relief (cough often has
an allergic basis and antihistamines are also thought
to reduce excessive secretions in the air passages).

What are some possible side effects?

Most patients taking this drug will not experience any
side effects. However, some patients who are sensitive
to one or another of the ingredients in Actifed-C
Expectorant may notice mild stimulation or sedation.
Since this drug contains two of the same ingredients as
Actifed (see above), similar side effects are possible.

What should you know about the drug?

The FDA, based partly on a review by the National
Academy of Sciences, states that Actifed-C Expectorant is "lacking substantial evidence of effectiveness
as a fixed combination" for the symptomatic relief of
cough in the following conditions: common cold, acute
bronchitis, allergic asthma, bronchiolitis, croup, emphysema, and tracheobronchitis.

Are there any special precautions?

The codeine ingredient in this drug may be habit-
forming.

   Actifed-C Expectorant should not be given to pregnant women, since its possible effect on a developing
fetus has not been established. It should be used with
caution in patients with high blood pressure (hypertension).

Aldactazide®

Generic name

This product contains a combination of spironolactone
and hydrochlorothiazide.

Class of drug
Diuretic and antihypertensive

In what form is the drug available?
Tablets

Why is the drug prescribed?
This product contains two ingredients which, acting together, have an additive effect in ridding the body of excessive amounts of water and salt (diuretic action) and in reducing high blood pressure (antihypertensive action). That is, the combined effect is greater than either ingredient used alone. The spironolactone ingredient in this combination (see Aldactone) tends to minimize the loss of the essential mineral potassium through the kidneys. This might occur if the hydrochlorothiazide component was prescribed alone.

Aldactazide is a potent drug and the manufacturer cautions that its unnecessary use should be avoided. It is recommended only in the treatment of the following conditions: congestive heart failure, cirrhosis of the liver, essential hypertension, and the nephrotic syndrome (a condition marked by high levels of protein in the urine, abnormally low levels of albumin in the blood, and excessive accumulation of water in the tissues).

What are some possible side effects?
Because one of the ingredients is the same as in Aldactone, similar side effects can occur with the use of Aldactazide. In addition, the more frequently encountered side effects include excessive thirst, weakness, restlessness, cramps or muscular pains, a drop in blood pressure (hypotension), and gastrointestinal symptoms such as nausea, vomiting, diarrhea, and abdominal cramps.

Less frequently, Aldactazide may cause the inability to achieve or maintain an erection of the penis (impotence), disorders of the blood-forming tissues (e.g., impairment of the ability of the bone marrow to manufacture white blood cells), inflammation of the pancreas (pancreatitis), a particular form of anemia (aplastic anemia), a diminished flow of urine from the kidneys (oliguria), and rapid beating of the heart (tachycardia). However, these side effects usually disappear once the use of Aldactazide is discontinued.

What should you know about the drug?

Aldactazide is not recommended as the initial treatment for fluid retention (edema) or high blood pressure. Any fixed-dose combination drug such as this must be carefully selected on its specific value for an individual patient.

Physicians have been warned about the unnecessary use of Aldactazide, since in experimental studies on rats one of its ingredients (spironolactone) has been shown to cause the development of tumors.

Are there any special precautions?

Aldactazide should not be taken by pregnant women, and its use in persons with impaired kidney function is not generally advised.

Aldactone®

Generic name
Spironolactone

Class of drug
Diuretic and antihypertensive

In what form is the drug available?
Tablets

Why is the drug prescribed?

It acts to eliminate the accumulation of excessive amounts of water and salt from the tissues (diuretic action) and to reduce high blood pressure (antihypertensive action). Water accumulation is one result of several disorders, including congestive heart failure, kidney disease, and cirrhosis of the liver. Although the drug helps the kidneys pass water and salt, it tends to spare the essential mineral potassium. Most other diuretics do not permit the retention of this mineral.

What are some possible side effects?

The more frequently encountered side effects include dry mouth, drowsiness, headache, skin rash, breast enlargement in males (gynecomastia), and irregular menstrual periods.

Because the drug does not flush out potassium through the kidneys, there is a possible danger of excessive potassium increase in the body. This is particularly true if a patient is taking supplementary doses of this mineral. Unchecked, this can lead to extremely serious side effects. Blood tests at intervals during therapy will alert a physician to any dangerous increase in the body's level of potassium.

What should you know about the drug?
Physicians have been warned about the unnecessary use of this drug, since in experimental studies in rats it has been shown to cause the development of tumors.

When taking the drug it is important not to take supplemental amounts of potassium or eat an excessive amount of foods rich in potassium.

Are there any special precautions?
Aldactone should not be taken by pregnant women, and its use in persons with impaired kidney function is not generally advised.

Aldomet®

Generic name
Methyldopa

Class of drug
Antihypertensive (hypotensive agent)

In what form is the drug available?
Tablets

Why is the drug prescribed?
This drug is used to reduce high blood pressure (hypertension). Exactly how this is achieved is somewhat unclear. But it is presumed that the drug reduces the ability of the nervous system to maintain a strong constricting effect on the blood vessels (vasoconstriction), which can be a cause of high blood pressure.

What are some possible side effects?
Among the more frequently encountered side effects are sedation, headache, weakness, dizziness, lightheadedness, nausea and vomiting, diarrhea, constipation, and mental disturbances including mild depression and nightmares.

Less frequently, the use of Aldomet may be associated with liver disorders (e.g., jaundice or hepatitis) and more severe disorders of the nervous system (e.g., Bell's palsy or Parkinsonism). It may also be responsible for inducing a drug-related fever.

In rare cases, Aldomet has been implicated as causing potentially fatal complications involving the liver and the blood-forming tissues (hemolytic anemia).

What should you know about the drug?

Physicians have been warned by the manufacturer to be alert for any complications that might occur during Aldomet therapy.

Are there any special precautions?

Aldomet should be used with extreme caution in patients with angina pectoris, an active disease of the liver, or a known history of liver disease.

Although there have been no unusual side effects reported in pregnant women undergoing Aldomet therapy, the possibility of injury to a developing fetus cannot be excluded. Also, the possibility of injury to a nursing infant cannot be excluded.

Aldoril®

Generic name

This product contains a combination of methyldopa and hydrochlorothiazide.

Class of drug

Antihypertensive and diuretic

In what form is the drug available?

Tablets

Why is the drug prescribed?

This combination product is designed to reduce high blood pressure (antihypertensive action) and eliminate the accumulation of excessive amounts of water and salt from the tissues (diuretic action). Both ingredients act to lower blood pressure in patients with hypertension. When taken together, they tend to produce a more effective antihypertensive response than either compound used alone.

Aldoril is especially useful in the treatment of high blood pressure when the retention of water and salt in the tissues is an underlying problem.

What are some possible side effects?

Because one of the ingredients is the same as in Aldomet (see above), similar side effects can occur with the use of Aldoril. Additional side effects may be related to the hydrochlorothiazide ingredient.

What should you know about the drug?

Aldoril is not recommended for the initial treatment of high blood pressure. Any fixed-dose combination drug such as this must be carefully selected according to its specific value for an individual patient.

Are there any special precautions?

The precautions to be considered in the use of this combination product are listed under Aldomet and hydrochlorothiazide.

Ambenyl® Expectorant

Generic name

This product contains a combination of codeine sulfate, bromodiphenhydramine hydrochloride, diphenhydramine hydrochloride, ammonium chloride, potassium guaiacolsulfonate, plus menthol and alcohol.

Class of drug

Antitussive and expectorant (plus antihistamines)

In what form is the drug available?

Syrup

Why is the drug prescribed?

It is designed to suppress coughs (antitussive action) and to loosen secretions in the air passages (expectorant action).

What are some possible side effects?

Among the more frequently encountered side effects are drowsiness, confusion, nervousness, restlessness, nausea and vomiting, diarrhea, constipation, blurred vision, and difficulty in urination. In susceptible individuals it can also cause the sensation of pounding of the heart (palpitations).

Less frequently the drug may cause a drop in blood pressure (hypotension), hives or a drug rash, and, in rare cases, a form of anemia (hemolytic anemia).

What should you know about the drug?

The manufacturer states that Ambenyl Expectorant is useful for control of coughs due to the common cold or allergies. However, the FDA, based partly on a review of the drug by the National Academy of Sciences, cautions that, "There is a lack of substantial evidence that this fixed combination drug has the effect purported."

Are there any special precautions?

Ambenyl Expectorant should not be given to persons with a known hypersensitivity (allergic reaction) to any of its ingredients.

The codeine ingredient of this product may be habit-forming.

While taking this drug, avoid using alcohol, tranquilizers, sedatives, or antihistamines which can have an additive effect on depressing the central nervous system and cause drowsiness or extreme tiredness.

Accidental ingestion or overdosage of this drug by children can be potentially fatal.

amoxicillin

Brand names

Amoxil® Larotid® Polymox® Robamox® Trimox® Wymox®

Class of drug

Broad-spectrum antibiotic (semisynthetic penicillin)

In what form is the drug available?

Capsules, liquid (oral suspension), and pediatric drops

Why is the drug prescribed?

It is used in the treatment of a fairly wide range of bacterial infections.

What are some possible side effects?

The more frequently encountered side effects include various types of skin rashes, nausea, vomiting, and diarrhea.

As with other drugs in this general group (the penicillins), amoxicillin can cause a disturbance of the normal bacterial population of the digestive tract. This promotes an overgrowth of one or more species of microorganisms. An example of the result of such a superinfection is inflammation of the lining of the mouth (stomatitis) and the tongue (glossitis).

What should you know about the drug?

Individuals who are allergic to penicillin should also be considered allergic to amoxicillin including, of course, all the brand names listed above. In such hypersensitive people the drug can cause a severe and potentially fatal reaction (anaphylactic shock).

As with all antibiotics, amoxicillin should be taken exactly as prescribed by your physician. Do not stop taking the drug just because you feel better. Complete the full course of therapy as directed on the label.

Are there any special precautions?

Amoxicillin should never be given to anyone with a known allergic reaction to it or to penicillin. There is also a greater chance that an adverse reaction will occur if the patient has a general history of other allergies such as hay fever, asthma, or hives.

ampicillin

Brand names

Alpen® Amcill® Omnipen® Pen-A® Penbritin® Pensyn® Polycillin® Principen® SK-Ampicillin® Totacillin®

Class of drug

Broad-spectrum antibiotic (semisynthetic penicillin)

In what form is the drug available?

Capsules and oral suspension (injectable form also available)

Why is the drug prescribed?

It is used in the treatment of a wide variety of bacterial infections, including those that involve the respiratory tract, urinary tract, gastrointestinal tract, the middle ear (otitis media), the skin, and the membranes that cover the brain (meningitis). The injectable form is used only for severe infections.

What are some possible side effects?

The most frequently encountered side effects are skin

rashes and diarrhea. Some patients have nausea, vomiting, and other signs that the digestive tract's normal bacterial population has been disturbed; this promotes overgrowth of one or more microorganism species. The result of this superinfection is inflammation of the lining of the mouth (stomatitis) and tongue (glossitis). Other side effects reported include anemia, high fever, otherwise unexplained bruising or unusual bleeding, and swelling and pain in the joints.

What should you know about the drug?

Individuals who are allergic to penicillin should also be considered allergic to ampicillin and, of course, any of the brand names listed above. In such hypersensitive people the drug can cause a severe and potentially fatal reaction (anaphylactic shock).

As with all antibiotics, ampicillin should be taken exactly as prescribed by your physician. Do not stop taking the drug just because you feel better. Complete the full course of therapy as directed on the label.

Are there any special precautions?

Ampicillin should never be given to anyone with a known allergic reaction to it or to penicillin. There is also a greater chance that an adverse reaction will occur if the patient has a general history of other allergies such as hay fever, asthma, or hives.

Patients with infectious mononucleosis (mono or glandular fever) should not take ampicillin. The incidence of skin rash in this group is very high.

Antivert®

Generic name
Meclizine

Class of drug
Antihistamine and antivertigo agent

In what form is the drug available?
Tablets and chewable tablets

Why is the drug prescribed?
It is used to prevent or control nausea, vomiting, and dizziness associated with motion sickness and disorders affecting the inner ear.

What are some possible side effects?

The most frequently encountered side effects are drowsiness, dryness of the mouth, and blurred vision.

What should you know about the drug?

The FDA, based partly on a review of this drug by the National Academy of Sciences, states that Antivert is "effective" in the management of nausea and vomiting, and dizziness associated with motion sickness. They also state that the drug is "possibly effective" in the management of vertigo associated with diseases affecting the vestibular system (inner ear).

Are there any special precautions?

This drug should not be given to pregnant women or to women who are likely to become pregnant.

Apresoline® Hydrochloride

Generic name
Hydralazine hydrochloride

Class of drug
Antihypertensive

In what form is the drug available?
Tablets (an injectable form is also available)

Why is the drug prescribed?
It is used, alone or in combination with other drugs, to reduce high blood pressure (hypertension). Most commonly, it is prescribed to treat a specific form of high blood pressure known as essential hypertension where the underlying cause of the elevated blood pressure is not known and an associated disease of the kidneys does not exist.

What are some possible side effects?
The most frequently encountered side effects include headaches, nausea and vomiting, diarrhea, an abnormally rapid heartbeat (tachycardia), and a sensation of the heartbeat which is usually not associated with an increase in the heart rate (palpitations). Some patients also have experienced an attack of angina pectoris (a sudden pain in the chest caused by a temporarily insufficient supply of blood to the heart muscle).

Less frequently encountered side effects include dizziness, vertigo, muscle cramps, tremors, conjunctivitis, depression, anxiety, and drug-induced skin rashes (an allergic reaction).

In a few cases the drug has impaired the ability of the blood-forming tissues to manufacture red and white blood cells. Reports also exist that some patients, while taking Apresoline, have experienced a paradoxical response in which the blood pressure, instead of being lowered, goes even higher.

What should you know about the drug?

Overdosage with this potent drug can cause a severe disturbance of the heartbeat (cardiac arrhythmia), and shock which can be fatal unless immediate medical treatment is available.

Experimental studies in mice have shown that Apresoline can cause certain birth defects such as cleft palate and malformations of facial and cranial bones in these animals. A direct effect on a human fetus has not been shown. However, because of the possible risk, Apresoline is not generally recommended for use during pregnancy.

Are there any special precautions?

Apresoline should be used with extreme caution (if at all) during pregnancy. Its use alone is also not generally recommended in patients with suspected disease of the heart, or the coronary arteries that supply blood to the heart muscle. In patients with advanced disease of the kidneys, the use of Apresoline requires special precautions.

Atarax®

Generic name
Hydroxyzine hydrochloride

Class of drug
Minor tranquilizer (antianxiety agent) and antiemetic

In what form is the drug available?
Tablets and syrup

Why is the drug prescribed?

It is used primarily in the treatment of emotional stress or disturbances characterized by anxiety, tension, apprehension, agitation, or confusion.

Atarax is also used to control nausea and vomiting (antiemetic action).

What are some possible side effects?

No serious side effects have been reported. Drowsiness often occurs at the recommended doses and at high doses, the mouth may become dry.

What should you know about the drug?

The drug commonly exerts a calming effect within fifteen to thirty minutes following administration.

The dosage given varies widely with the individual requirement, and is usually adjusted during therapy according to the patient's response.

Are there any special precautions?

The drug should not be given during pregnancy, since its possible effect on the developing fetus has not yet been established. The drug has been shown to cause fetal abnormalities in mice, rats, and rabbits.

The effect of Atarax is increased if taken together with central nervous system depressants such as barbiturates or sleeping pills.

Atarax can cause drowsiness. Avoid any activity that demands mental alertness, such as driving a car or operating potentially dangerous machinery, until its effects on an individual patient are known.

Atromid-S®

Generic name
Clofibrate

Class of drug
Antilipidemic agent (reduces elevated serum lipids)

In what form is the drug available?
Capsules

Why is the drug prescribed?

It is used primarily to reduce high levels of cholesterol in the blood circulation. A high level of cholesterol in the blood has traditionally been considered significant as an index for predicting if an individual patient is at risk of a heart attack. (Cholesterol is a fatlike substance. It is found in the material that can clog or narrow the internal diameter of arteries in the condition known as atherosclerosis.)

What are some possible side effects?

The most frequently encountered side effects include nausea, vomiting, loose stools, abdominal distress, headache, dizziness, weakness, muscular cramps, itching, and skin rash. Some patients taking Atromid-S have experienced flulike symptoms, hair loss (alopecia), dry brittle hair, and dry skin.

Occasionally more serious side effects occur. These include: a disturbance of the heartbeat (cardiac arrhythmia), inflammation of the veins (phlebitis), and disorders of the blood. Some men may also experience a loss of sex drive and the inability to achieve and maintain an erection of the penis (impotence).

What should you know about the drug?

It is not clear if Atromid-S has any effect on preventing a heart attack by lowering the blood levels of cholesterol. It will take several years for researchers to discover the effectiveness of this drug.

Are there any special precautions?

Atromid-S should not be taken by pregnant women or those who are likely to become pregnant. Use of the drug should be discontinued several months before conception, in the case of a planned pregnancy.

Before prescribing this drug, physicians have been cautioned by the manufacturer to make every attempt to control a patient's blood levels of cholesterol by other means and by appropriate changes in diet.

Extreme caution must be taken when Atromid-S is given at the same time as anticoagulants (drugs which tend to keep the blood from clotting). This is advised to prevent the possibility of bleeding complications.

Azo Gantrisin®

Generic name
This product is a combination of sulfisoxazole and phenazopyridine hydrochloride.

Class of drug

Antibacterial (sulfonamide) and urinary analgesic

In what form is the drug available?

Tablets

Why is the drug prescribed?

It is used to treat infections and pain in the urinary tract. The sulfisoxazole ingredient acts to inhibit the growth and multiplication of certain species of bacteria. The phenazopyridine ingredient acts specifically to relieve the pain and burning sensation that often accompanies infections of the urinary tract (e.g., cystitis, pyelonephritis, and pyelitis).

What are some possible side effects?

The more frequently encountered side effects include nausea, vomiting, headache, abdominal pains, diarrhea, depression, and a ringing or hissing sensation in the ears (tinnitus).

Less frequently encountered side effects include impairment of the blood-forming tissues (e.g., certain forms of anemia and interference with the ability of the bone marrow to manufacture red and white blood cells), allergic reactions (e.g., skin rashes, joint pain, and inflammation of the heart muscle), inflammation of the liver (hepatitis), and inflammation of the pancreas (pancreatitis).

Some patients taking Azo Gantrisin have also experienced convulsions and severe allergic (anaphylactoid) reactions.

What should you know about the drug?

Azo Gantrisin contains a sulfonamide (sulfa drug). The administration of drugs in this class has been associated with deaths from severe hypersensitivity (allergic) reactions. In addition, symptoms such as sore throat, fever, pallor, purpura or jaundice may be early signs of serious blood disorders. Complete blood counts should frequently be performed on patients undergoing treatment with sulfonamides.

The phenazopyridine ingredient in Azo Gantrisin colors the urine orange-red. This occurs soon after taking the drug, but is absolutely harmless.

Are there any special precautions?

The safe use of sulfonamides by pregnant women has

26

not been established. Experimental studies in mice
and rats reveal that the drug causes congenital malformations in the offspring of these animals including
cleft palate and other bone abnormalities.

Azo Gantrisin must not be taken by a pregnant
woman at term or during the nursing period. Sulfonamides pass the placenta and are excreted in the mother's milk and may cause kernicterus (a serious form of
jaundice) in the nursing infant.

Bactrim®

Generic name
This product contains a combination of trimethoprim
and sulfamethoxazole.

Class of drug
Antibacterial

In what form is the drug available?
Tablets and oral suspension

Why is the drug prescribed?
It is used mainly to treat bacterial infections of the
urinary tract (kidneys and bladder).

Bactrim also is used in the treatment of certain
other bacterial infections, including inflammation of
the middle ear (acute otitis media).

What are some possible side effects?
The most frequently encountered side effects include
nausea, vomiting, abdominal pain, diarrhea, headache,
and skin rashes.

Some patients taking Bactrim may experience
drug-induced fever, chills, inflammation of the mouth
(stomatitis) or tongue (glossitis), and difficulty urinating.

A few patients may also have mental depression, a
ringing in the ears (tinnitus), vertigo, insomnia, inflammation of the liver (hepatitis), severe allergic
reactions (anaphylactic shock), and impairment of the
blood-forming tissues.

What should you know about the drug?
The manufacturer warns that Bactrim should *not* be
used in the treatment of strep throat.

One of the ingredients of Bactrim is a sulfonamide or sulfa drug (sulfamethoxazole). Such drugs should be given with caution to patients with impaired function of the kidneys or liver, bronchial asthma, or severe allergies.

Are there any special precautions?

Drink plenty of water while being treated with Bactrim. This helps prevent the formation of crystals of the drug, which could form stones and damage the kidneys.

Discontinue the use of Bactrim and consult your physician immediately at the first sign of skin rashes, sore throat, pallor, or yellowness of the skin.

Bactrim should not be used during pregnancy or during the nursing period.

Consult your physician before taking any other drugs at the same time as Bactrim.

Benadryl®

Generic name
Diphenhydramine hydrochloride

Class of drug
Antihistamine

In what form is the drug available?
Tablets and elixir (an injectable form is also available)

Why is the drug prescribed?
The main use of this drug is to relieve symptoms of various allergies, including hay fever (allergic rhinitis), allergic conjunctivitis, and hives (urticaria). It is also used to prevent or relieve the symptoms of motion sickness.

Less common uses of Benadryl include the treatment of mild cases of Parkinsonism, and as part of the follow-up treatment of severe allergic reactions (anaphylactic shock).

What are some possible side effects?
The most frequently encountered side effects include sedation, sleepiness, dizziness, disturbed coordination, abdominal distress, and thickening of the bronchial secretions.

Less frequently encountered side effects include: headache; hives (urticaria); drug rash; sensitivity to light (photosensitivity); excessive perspiration; chills; dryness of the mouth, nose, and throat; nausea and vomiting; diarrhea; constipation; nervousness; irritability; restlessness; blurred vision; ringing in the ears (tinnitus); stuffy nose; wheezing; and difficulty urinating. Some patients experience a drop in blood pressure (hypotension), rapid heartbeat (tachycardia), and a sensation of a rapid heartbeat (palpitations).

A few patients, while taking Benadryl, have had anemia and other disorders of the blood. Rare cases have also been reported of severe allergic reactions (anaphylactic shock).

What should you know about the drug?

Elderly persons are especially prone to experience dizziness, sedation, and a drop in blood pressure while taking antihistamines such as Benadryl.

The dosage of Benadryl must be adapted to the needs and therapeutic response of the individual patient. Overdosage can cause either stimulation or depression of the central nervous system, which requires immediate medical attention. Children are particularly likely to experience stimulation.

Are there any special precautions?

Benadryl should not be given to newborn or premature infants, or to nursing mothers.

The depressant effect of Benadryl on the central nervous system is increased by taking alcohol, sedatives, sleeping pills, or tranquilizers.

Benadryl, as well as other antihistamines, must be used with caution in persons with a particular form of glaucoma (narrow-angle glaucoma), obstruction of the neck of the bladder, peptic ulcer, and obstruction of the passage between the stomach and the small intestine (pyloroduodenal obstruction).

Overdosage in infants or children may cause convulsions or death.

Bendectin®

Generic name

This product contains a combination of doxylamine succinate and pyridoxine hydrochloride.

Class of drug
Antihistamine (with antiemetic action) and vitamin B_6

In what form is the drug available?
Tablets

Why is the drug prescribed?
It is used to prevent or relieve symptoms of nausea and vomiting during pregnancy (morning sickness).

What are some possible side effects?
The doxylamine succinate ingredient (an antihistamine) may cause the following side effects: drowsiness, vertigo, nervousness, abdominal pain, headache, a sensation of the heartbeat (palpitations), diarrhea, disorientation, or irritability. The pyridoxine hydrochloride ingredient (vitamin B_6) is not known to cause any adverse reactions.

What should you know about the drug?
Bendectin appears to be relatively safe for use by pregnant women. However, substantial proof does not exist that the pyridoxine hydrochloride ingredient contributes significantly to the intended effect of this combination product.

Are there any special precautions?
Bendectin may cause drowsiness. Thus, it should be used with caution when driving or operating dangerous machinery.

Bentyl® with Phenobarbital

Generic name
Dicyclomine hydrochloride plus phenobarbital

Class of drug
Anticholinergic (antispasmodic) and sedative

In what form is the drug available?
Capsules, tablets, and syrup

Why is the drug prescribed?
It is used primarily to relieve the symptoms of intestinal spasm associated with certain disorders of the gastrointestinal tract.

What are some possible side effects?

The most frequently encountered side effects are drowsiness and blurred vision. Other reported side effects include: retention of urine, rapid heartbeat (tachycardia), a sensation of the heartbeat (palpitations), headache, nervousness, dizziness, insomnia, nausea and vomiting, dilation of the pupils, the inability to achieve or maintain an erection of the penis (impotence), suppression of the flow of breast milk (lactation), constipation, skin rashes or hives (urticaria), and a bloated feeling. Some patients have experienced severe allergic reactions (anaphylactic shock).

What should you know about the drug?

The phenobarbital ingredient in Bentyl may be habit-forming. In certain cases the abrupt withdrawal of the drug may cause delirium or convulsions.

Bentyl can cause a reduction in the ability to sweat. Thus, its use in hot climates may lead to heat prostration (heat stroke) and fever.

Are there any special precautions?

Bentyl should be used with caution in patients with glaucoma, disease of the prostate gland, disease of the liver or kidneys, ulcerative colitis, hyperthyroidism, heart disease, and high blood pressure.

Butazolidin® Alka

Generic name

This product contains a combination of phenylbutazone, dried aluminum hydroxide gel, and magnesium trisilicate.

Class of drug

Antiarthritic and anti-inflammatory agent (plus antacids)

In what form is the drug available?

Capsules

Why is the drug prescribed?

It is used to provide symptomatic relief of pain and disability associated with a wide variety of severe inflammation of the joints. These include: gout (or gouty arthritis), rheumatoid arthritis, rheumatoid spondylitis, osteoarthritis, psoriatic arthritis, and painful shoulder (e.g., bursitis of the shoulder).

The drug is also used in the relief of certain forms of vein inflammation (superficial thrombophlebitis).

What are some possible side effects?

This extremely potent drug can cause a variety of side effects. However, because Butazolidin *cannot cure* disease of the joints—it only provides symptomatic relief—the potentially serious and sometimes fatal side effects do not justify its routine use.

The phenylbutazone ingredient of this drug is capable of impairing the manufacturing of red and white blood cells by the bone marrow. This occasionally leads to fatal complications such as agranulocytosis, aplastic anemia, and hemolytic anemia.

Among other serious side effects reported with the use of Butazolidin are: leukemia, fatal and nonfatal inflammation of the liver (hepatitis), severe allergic reactions (anaphylactic shock), kidney failure, high blood pressure (hypertension), detached retina, hearing loss, convulsions, hallucinations, and psychosis.

What should you know about the drug?

Physicians have been warned that patients receiving Butazolidin should be given blood tests throughout therapy at intervals of one or, at most, two weeks. This is in addition to other special tests pertinent to the individual patient.

Are there any special precautions?

Butazolidin is not a drug for casual use. It can be extremely toxic. Patients taking the product should report any adverse effects to their physician immediately. Do not take Butazolidin without a physician's knowledge. Adverse effects may occur.

Butisol Sodium®

Generic name
Sodium butabarbital

Class of drug
Sedative and hypnotic (sleep-inducing drug)

In what form is the drug available?
Tablets and elixir

Why is the drug prescribed?
Butisol, which acts to depress the activity of the central nervous system, is used primarily in the treatment of insomnia, to relieve anxiety, and to provide sedation prior to a surgical procedure.

What are some possible side effects?
Possible side effects with the use of this drug include depression of the nerve centers that control breathing (respiratory depression), depression of the central nervous system, shock, nausea and vomiting, skin rash, the effect of a drug hangover, and paradoxical excitement (the opposite drug action intended).

What should you know about the drug?
Butisol may impair mental alertness and limit the ability to perform potentially hazardous tasks. These include driving and operating machinery.

The use of alcohol or other depressants of the central nervous system while taking Butisol may add to the sedative effects of the drug.

The prolonged use of drugs in this class may result in dependence on the particular drug. Withdrawal symptoms may occur and finally result in delirium, convulsions, or death.

Are there any special precautions?
Butisol should not be given to persons who are sensitive to barbiturates. It should also not be given to patients with porphyria (any of a group of rare metabolic disorders involving the complex chemical compounds known as prophrins).

Catapres®

Generic name
Clonidine hydrochloride

Class of drug
Antihypertensive

In what form is the drug available?
Tablets

Why is the drug prescribed?

It is used, often in combination with certain other drugs, to reduce high blood pressure (hypertension).

What are some possible side effects?

The most frequently encountered side effects are dry mouth, drowsiness, and sedation. Less frequently encountered side effects include constipation, dizziness, headache, and fatigue. In continued therapy with Catapres, these side effects often tend to diminish.

A few patients taking Catapres have experienced nausea, vomiting, loss of appetite (anorexia), weight gain, insomnia, and various mental and behavioral changes.

What should you know about the drug?

When therapy with Catapres is to be discontinued, the dose should be gradually reduced over a period of two to four days. Abrupt discontinuation of the drug can cause a severe rise in blood pressure, nervousness, agitation, and headache.

The sedative effects of Catapres can be increased by taking alcohol, tranquilizers, or other substances that depress the central nervous system. Use caution when driving, operating potentially dangerous machinery, or engaging in other tasks that demand mental alertness.

Are there any special precautions?

Patients undergoing long-term therapy with Catapres should have periodic eye examinations. Experimental studies in animals have shown that the drug can cause degeneration of the retina in rats.

Do not discontinue the use of Catapres without first consulting your physician. Otherwise, severe side effects can occur. Catapres should be used with extreme caution (if at all) during pregnancy.

Chlor-Trimeton®

Generic name

This product is a combination of chlorpheniramine maleate and pseudoephedrine sulfate.

Class of drug

Antihistamine and decongestant

In what form is the drug available?
Tablets

Why is the drug prescribed?
It is used to provide temporary relief from the symptoms of hay fever (allergic rhinitis) and other allergies that affect the upper respiratory tract. It helps relieve nasal congestion, runny nose, sneezing, itchy or watery eyes, and sinus congestion.

What are some possible side effects?
The most frequently encountered side effect is drowsiness. Some persons, especially children, may experience excitability.

Other side effects are less frequent. They include: dizziness, vertigo, disturbed coordination, a ringing in the ears (tinnitus), restlessness, and insomnia.

What should you know about the drug?
Patients are cautioned that the effects of Chlor-Trimeton are increased by taking alcohol, sedatives, tranquilizers, or other substances that depress the central nervous system.

This drug may impair mental alertness. Thus, until its effects on an individual are known, it is best not to drive, operate machinery, or perform any other potentially hazardous task.

Are there any special precautions?
Chlor-Trimeton must be used cautiously in patients with high blood pressure (hypertension), heart disease, asthma, glaucoma, overactive thyroid gland (hyperthyroidism), disease of the prostate, and diabetes.

Combid®

Generic name
This product contains a combination of prochlorperazine and isopropamide iodide.

Class of drug
Anticholinergic (antispasmodic) and antinauseant

In what form is the drug available?
Capsules

Why is the drug prescribed?

It is used to prevent or inhibit painful spasms of the stomach and intestines and control nausea and vomiting. Combid also reduces the secretion of stomach juices and relieves anxiety and tension.

What are some possible side effects?

The more frequently encountered side effects include dry mouth, retention of urine, rapid heartbeat (tachycardia), sensation of the heartbeat (palpitations), dilation of the pupils, blurred vision, constipation, nausea, stuffy nose, a bloated feeling, and drug-induced fever.

Occasionally, more serious side effects are reported. These include: convulsions, a severe and sometimes fatal drop in blood pressure, cardiac arrest (a sudden loss of heart function, resulting in cessation of the blood circulation), and disorders of the blood-forming tissues.

Numerous other side effects are reported by the manufacturer. Many are related to individual patient sensitivity, while others appear to occur particularly in patients with special medical problems.

What should you know about the drug?

The FDA, based partly on a review of the drug by the National Academy of Sciences, states that Combid is "possibly effective as adjunctive therapy in peptic ulcer and in the irritable bowel syndrome (irritable colon, spastic colon, mucous colitis, functional gastrointestinal disorders), and functional diarrhea."

Combid should be used with caution (if at all) during pregnancy. This class of drug may also inhibit the flow of breast milk during the period of lactation.

The effects of Combid are increased by taking alcohol, sedatives, tranquilizers, or other substances that depress the central nervous system. Patients are thus cautioned about activities that require mental alertness such as driving or operating potentially dangerous machinery.

Are there any special precautions?

Combid should be used cautiously (if at all) in persons with a known history of jaundice, liver disease, or disorders of the blood. If any of these disorders are still active, the drug should not be prescribed.

In addition, Combid should not be used in persons

with glaucoma, obstruction of the passage between the stomach and small intestines (pyloric obstruction), disease of the prostate gland, or obstruction of the neck of the bladder.

Combid should not be given to children under the age of twelve.

Compazine®

Generic name
Prochlorperazine

Class of drug
Major tranquilizer (antipsychotic) and antinauseant

In what form is the drug available?
Tablets, capsules, and suppositories (an injectable form is also available)

Why is the drug prescribed?
It is used in the treatment of severe emotional disorders (psychoses) to relieve anxiety and tension. Compazine is also used to control severe nausea and vomiting.

What are some possible side effects?
The most frequently encountered side effects include drowsiness, dizziness, absence or abnormal cessation of the menstrual periods (amenorrhea), blurred vision, skin reactions, and a drop in blood pressure (hypotension). Some patients, while taking Compazine, have had jaundice and impairment of the blood-forming tissues.

This class of drug can also cause various neuromuscular reactions. These include spasms of the neck muscles, rigidity of the back muscles, difficulty in swallowing, tremors, and convulsions.

Occasionally, patients taking drugs in the class of phenothiazine derivatives, which includes Compazine, have experienced a severe and sometimes fatal drop in blood pressure, and cardiac arrest (a sudden loss of heart function, resulting in cessation of the blood circulation).

What should you know about the drug?
Children with illnesses such as chicken pox, measles,

inflammation of the intestinal tract (gastroenteritis), infections of the central nervous system, or dehydration seem to be much more susceptible to neuromuscular reactions than are adults. In such patients, the drug should be used only under close medical supervision.

The effects of Compazine are increased by taking alcohol, sedatives, tranquilizers, or other substances that depress the central nervous system. Patients are thus cautioned about performing activities that require mental alertness such as driving or operating potentially dangerous machinery.

Are there any special precautions?

The safe use of Compazine during pregnancy has not been established. It should therefore be used only if the therapeutic benefits clearly outweigh the possible risk of injury to the developing fetus. The drug should never be taken by children under the age of twelve.

Cordran®

Generic name
Flurandrenolide

Class of drug
Corticosteroid

In what form is the drug available?
Cream, ointment, and lotion

Why is the drug prescribed?
It is used topically (on the skin surface) to treat various inflammatory skin disorders.

What are some possible side effects?

The most frequently encountered side effects with the use of any topical corticosteroids including Cordran are itching, dry skin, a burning sensation, and skin eruptions. These occur at the site where the drug is applied. They are more common when a tight dressing is placed over the affected area of skin.

If Cordran is applied to a wide area of the body for prolonged periods, the drug may be absorbed through the skin and cause additional problems, some of which are potentially serious.

What should you know about the drug?

If Cordran causes local skin irritation, its use should be discontinued.

Skin infections do not respond to Cordran. In such cases an appropriate antibacterial or antifungal agent should first be used to clear the infection. Applying Cordran may cause the infection to spread.

Are there any special precautions?

Use Cordran only under the close supervision of your physician. Do not apply the drug to areas of the skin that seem infected.

The safe use of Cordran during pregnancy has not been established.

Cortisporin® Otic

Generic name
This product contains a combination of polymyxin B sulfate, neomycin sulfate, and hydrocortisone.

Class of drug
Antibiotic and steroid

In what form is the drug available?
Liquid (applied with a dropper)

Why is the drug prescribed?
It is used to treat bacterial infections of the ear canal (external auditory canal).

What are some possible side effects?
Many people are sensitive to neomycin, one of the antibiotic ingredients of Cortisporin Otic. The drug may cause the skin to become red and swollen. Itching and dry scaling of the skin may also occur.

If Cortisporin Otic reaches the middle ear (located just behind the eardrum), as in cases of perforated eardrum, it can cause stinging and burning.

What should you know about the drug?
Cortisporin Otic contains a combination of two antibiotics to treat bacterial infection, and a steroid drug to relieve inflammation of the affected tissues of the ear canal. Prolonged use of this, or any antibiotic, may result in the local overgrowth of certain nonsusceptible

microorganisms (e.g., various species of fungi). Physicians have been advised to discontinue the use of Cortisporin Otic if the ear infection has not improved within one week.

Are there any special precautions?

The use of Cortisporin Otic should be discontinued if it causes local irritation, or if there is other evidence of sensitivity.

If the solution is warmed before use, take care that it is not heated above normal body temperature (98.6°F., 37.0°C), as this could affect its potency.

Coumadin®

Generic name
Crystalline warfarin sodium

Class of drug
Anticoagulant

In what form is the drug available?
Tablets

Why is the drug prescribed?

It is used in the treatment or prevention of blood clots (anticoagulation). A thrombus occurs when the clot remains at its site of formation (thrombosis). An embolus occurs when the clot breaks away and is carried in the bloodstream until it obstructs a smaller vessel (embolism).

What are some possible side effects?

The principal side effect that can occur while taking Coumadin or other anticoagulants, is spontaneous bleeding. The bleeding may be minor or major, and can occur from any organ or tissue. The resulting signs and symptoms vary with the site of bleeding and its extent.

Other side effects are infrequent. They include: hair loss (alopecia), hives (urticaria), skin inflammation (dermatitis), nausea, diarrhea, abdominal cramps, and fever.

What should you know about the drug?

The risk of bleeding while taking an anticoagulant,

such as Coumadin, is minimized by carefully adjusting the dosage to the needs of an individual patient. The physician's instructions must be followed precisely.

Are there any special precautions?
Coumadin is a potent drug with a narrow margin between desired therapeutic effect (thinning of the blood) and the risk of spontaneous bleeding. Some other drugs, if taken at the same time as Coumadin, can cause potentially serious complications. Thus, it is essential that you tell your physician what other drugs you have been taking so he or she can advise which you may continue to take. These include aspirin and other products that do not require a prescription (over-the-counter drugs).

Any signs of bleeding while taking Coumadin should be reported to your physician immediately. These include: bleeding from the mouth or gums, red or dark brown urine, spitting or coughing up of blood, nosebleed, excessive menstrual flow, and unexplained bruising of the skin (black and blue marks).

Cyclospasmol®

Generic name
Cyclandelate

Class of drug
Vasodilator

In what form is the drug available?
Capsules and tablets

Why is the drug prescribed?
It is used to relieve symptoms of an inadequate blood supply to the extremities, including the hands and feet (peripheral vascular disease).

Cyclospasmol also is used to relieve symptoms associated with an inadequate supply of blood to the brain (cerebral vascular insufficiency).

The drug is designed to achieve its effects by relaxing the blood vessels, thus permitting an increased flow of blood.

What are some possible side effects?
The most frequently encountered side effects are

heartburn (pyrosis), abdominal pain or discomfort, flushing, headache, weakness, and an increase in the heart rate (tachycardia).

What should you know about the drug?

The American Medical Association, in their publication *AMA Drug Evaluations*, states: "The place of this agent [Cyclospasmol] in therapy has not been clearly established."

The FDA, based partly on a review of the drug by the National Academy of Sciences, states that Cyclospasmol is "possibly effective" for the symptomatic relief of the vascular disorders listed by the manufacturer.

Are there any special precautions?

Cyclospasmol should be used with extreme caution in patients with heart disease, disease of the blood vessels of the brain, and glaucoma.

The safe use of this drug during pregnancy has not been established.

Dalmane®

Generic name
Flurazepam hydrochloride

Class of drug
Hypnotic agent (sleep-inducing drug)

In what form is the drug available?
Capsules

Why is the drug prescribed?
Dalmane is prescribed as a sleeping pill. It is useful in persons who have difficulty falling asleep, who wake up frequently during the night, or who continually awake too early in the morning.

What are some possible side effects?
This drug may cause lightheadedness, dizziness, depression, loss of coordination (staggering), and the feeling of having a hangover in the morning. Less frequently there have been reports of nausea, vomiting, diarrhea, severe sedation, headache, disorientation, apprehension, and body and joint pains.

What should you know about the drug?

The results of controlled studies suggest that this drug is able to induce sleep within an average of seventeen minutes and provides people who have had prior sleeping problems with an average of seven to eight hours sleep. Its sedative effects can be increased by alcohol and other drugs with a tranquilizing effect. This can be potentially dangerous, especially if driving, operating machinery, or performing any task that requires a high degree of mental alertness.

Prolonged use of this drug may result in psychological dependence.

Are there any special precautions?

This drug should not be taken by pregnant women, since there is some evidence that this general class of drug may cause birth defects.

Darvocet-N® 100

Generic name
This product contains a combination of propoxyphene napsylate and acetaminophen.

Class of drug
Analgesic

In what form is the drug available?
Tablets

Why is the drug prescribed?
It is used to relieve mild or moderate pain.

What are some possible side effects?
The most frequently encountered side effects include dizziness, sedation, nausea, and vomiting. In many cases these side effects can be alleviated if the patient lies down.

Less frequently encountered side effects include constipation, skin rashes, abdominal pain, lightheadedness, weakness, headache, minor visual disturbances, euphoria, and a feeling of unpleasantness or vague discomfort (dysphoria).

What should you know about the drug?
Darvocet-N 100 is a chemical derivative of methadone,

a narcotic painkiller, although it is not as potent. Death has occurred in some patients following overdose.

Are there any special precautions?
Darvocet-N 100 may impair mental alertness. Its effects are increased by taking alcohol, sedatives, tranquilizers, or other substances that depress the central nervous system. Caution must be used when driving or operating potentially dangerous machinery until the effects of the drug on a particular individual are known.

The use of this drug may cause psychological or physical dependence.

Darvocet-N 100 must be used with extreme caution (if at all) during pregnancy.

Darvon®

Generic name
Propoxyphene hydrochloride

Class of drug
Analgesic

In what form is the drug available?
Capsules

Why is the drug prescribed?
It is used to relieve mild or moderate pain.

What are some possible side effects?
The most frequently encountered side effects include dizziness, sedation, nausea, and vomiting. In many cases, these side effects can be alleviated if the patient lies down.

Less frequently encountered side effects include constipation, skin rashes, abdominal pain, lightheadedness, weakness, headache, minor visual disturbances, euphoria, and a feeling of unpleasantness or vague discomfort (dysphoria).

What should you know about the drug?
The results of some tests have suggested that taking Darvon may be no more effective than the psychological benefit of taking a sugar pill (placebo). The main

criticism is that the cost and potential side effects of Darvon may not justify its widespread use, compared with other analgesics (e.g., aspirin).

The long-term use of Darvon in very large doses (above 800 mg per day) has caused severe mental disturbances (psychoses) and convulsions. Death has occurred in some patients following overdose.

Are there any special precautions?

Darvon may impair mental alertness. Its effects are increased by taking alcohol, sedatives, tranquilizers, or other substances that depress the central nervous system. Caution must be taken when driving or operating potentially dangerous machinery until the effects of the drug on a particular individual are known.

The use of this drug may cause psychological or physical dependence.

Darvon must be used with extreme caution (if at all) during pregnancy.

Darvon® Compound-65

Generic name
This product contains a combination of propoxyphene hydrochloride, aspirin, phenacetin, and caffeine.

Class of drug
Analgesic

In what form is the drug available?
Capsules

Why is the drug prescribed?
It is used to relieve mild or moderate pain.

What are some possible side effects?
The most frequently encountered side effects include dizziness, sedation, nausea, and vomiting. In many cases these side effects can be alleviated if the patient lies down.

Less frequently encountered side effects include constipation, skin rashes, abdominal pain, lightheadedness, weakness, headache, minor visual disturbances, euphoria, and a feeling of unpleasantness or vague discomfort (dysphoria).

What should you know about the drug?

Darvon Compound-65 contains three painkillers (analgesics) plus a mild stimulant (caffeine). These ingredients are claimed to act together to provide a greater degree of pain relief than would any of the ingredients taken separately.

The long-term use of the propoxyphene hydrochloride ingredient of this product in very large doses has caused severe mental disturbances (psychoses) and convulsions. Death has occurred in some patients following overdose.

Are there any special precautions?

The aspirin ingredient of this product can cause stomach irritation or bleeding. This is especially a risk if the drug is taken in excessive amounts or over prolonged periods. Aspirin or products that contain aspirin, including Darvon Compound-65, must be used with extreme caution (if at all) by persons with peptic ulcer or blood-clotting abnormalities.

Darvon Compound-65 may impair mental alertness. Its effects are increased by taking alcohol, sedatives, tranquilizers, or other substances that depress the central nervous system. Caution must be taken when driving or operating potentially dangerous machinery until the effects of the drug on a particular individual are known.

The use of this drug may cause psychological or physical dependence.

Darvon Compound-65 must be used with extreme caution (if at all) during pregnancy.

Demulen®

Generic name

This product contains a combination of ethynodiol diacetate and ethinyl estradiol.

Class of drug

Oral contraceptive

In what form is the drug available?

Tablets

Why is the drug prescribed?

It is used to prevent pregnancy (contraception).

What are some possible side effects?

The most frequently encountered side effects that may result from the use of oral contraceptives are: nausea, bloating, vaginal bleeding, abdominal cramps, tenderness of the breasts, headache, vaginal itching, increased vaginal discharge, infection of the vagina, depression, fatigue, increased appetite, and weight gain.

In some instances, potentially more serious side effects can occur. These include: the formation of blood clots in deep veins, high blood pressure, gall bladder disease, and an increase in the blood sugar level.

Other serious diseases (e.g., breast cancer) are possibly related to taking oral contraceptives, but a clear cause-and-effect relationship remains to be proved.

What should you know about the drug?

Demulen, like many oral contraceptives, contains a combination of two synthetic female hormones. Acting together, they inhibit the release of new eggs from the ovary. Thus, ovulation is prevented and pregnancy is avoided. All modern oral contraceptives are extremely effective.

Are there any special precautions?

The manufacturer cautions that oral contraceptives should not be used in women with blood-clotting disorders, thrombophlebitis, heart disease, disease of the blood vessels of the brain (cerebral vascular disease), coronary artery disease, or in those with a history of these diseases or of myocardial infarction.

Oral contraceptives are not to be given to women with known or suspected breast cancer, undiagnosed vaginal bleeding, known or suspected pregnancy, or certain forms of liver disease.

Smoking cigarettes increases the risk of serious side effects while taking oral contraceptives. This risk increases both with age (especially in women over thirty-five) and the number of cigarettes smoked daily.

Diabinese®

Generic name
Chlorpropamide

Class of drug
Oral hypoglycemic (antidiabetic) agent

In what form is the drug available?
Tablets

Why is the drug prescribed?
It is used in the treatment of selected patients with diabetes; usually those with a relatively mild form of the disease. The majority of patients able to benefit from this class of drug (which is *not* insulin) experience the first signs of diabetes toward middle age (maturity-onset diabetes). The drug is of no value if the patient's pancreas is unable to manufacture insulin.

What are some possible side effects?
The most frequently encountered side effect is a severe *drop* in the level of sugar (glucose) in the blood. This condition is known as hypoglycemia. The patient becomes confused, weak, dizzy, and may break out in a cold sweat. In severe cases which require immediate medical attention, the patient may lapse into a coma.

Less frequently encountered side effects include abnormalities of the blood or liver, skin rashes, and retention of water in the tissues which causes swelling (edema).

What should you know about the drug?
A potentially dangerous drop in the level of blood sugar may occur if Diabinese is taken together with certain other drugs. These include: antibacterial sulfonamides, phenylbutazone, salicylates (e.g., aspirin), probenecid, dicoumarol, and MAO inhibitors.

Thiazide diuretics (water pills) may reduce the effects of Diabinese.

Diabinese should not be used to treat juvenile or growth-onset diabetes, severe or unstable (brittle) diabetes, or diabetes accompanied by various complications.

The drug should not be given to patients about to undergo major surgery, those with severe infections, or those who have suffered severe injuries.

Are there any special precautions?
If any side effects are experienced while taking Diabinese, consult your physician immediately.

digoxin

Brand names
Lanoxin® SK-Digoxin®

Class of drug
Cardiotonic glycoside (digitalis preparation obtained from the leaves of *Digitalis lanata)*

In what form is the drug available?
Tablets (also available are a liquid for injection and a pediatric elixir for children to be taken by mouth)

Why is the drug prescribed?
It is used in patients with certain types of heart disease to increase the force of contraction of the heart muscle and to control disorders of heart rhythm (irregular heartbeats).

What are some possible side effects?
The most frequently encountered side effects—especially early in the course of therapy when dosage is being adjusted by the physician for maximum effectiveness—include loss of appetite (anorexia), nausea, vomiting, and diarrhea. Some patients also experience visual disturbances (such as blurred vision or impaired perception of color), headache, drowsiness, confusion, and various kinds of skin rash or hives. Very large doses may cause convulsions and coma.

Less frequently, this drug has been implicated as the cause of disturbances in the normal heartbeat (cardiac arrhythmias).

What should you know about the drug?
Physicians have been warned not to use this drug in the treatment of excess body weight (obesity). This is a misuse of an extremely powerful drug, whose potential side effects, especially the disturbance of heart rhythm, can be severe.

Are there any special precautions?
This potent drug has a relatively narrow margin between therapeutic and toxic effects and should be taken exactly as prescribed.

Any side effects, no matter how minor, should be reported to your physician immediately to permit adjustment of the dosage.

Dilantin®

Generic name

Phenytoin (formerly known as diphenylhydantoin) sodium

Class of drug

Antiepileptic (anticonvulsant)

In what form is the drug available?

Capsules, tablets, and suspension (an injectable form is also available)

Why is the drug prescribed?

It is used mainly in patients with epilepsy to prevent seizures or reduce the frequency of convulsive attacks.

What are some possible side effects?

The most frequently encountered side effects include impaired muscular coordination, difficulty in walking, constant involuntary movement of the eyeballs (nystagmus), slurred speech, and mental confusion. These effects are often related to the amount of drug taken and may disappear at a reduced dosage level.

Other side effects include dizziness, insomnia, headache, nausea, vomiting, constipation, and skin rashes (more common in children). Swelling of the gums occurs frequently. It can often be prevented by good oral hygiene, including gum massage and frequent brushing.

Patients receiving Dilantin have occasionally experienced much more serious side effects. These include severe allergic skin reactions and impairment of the blood-forming tissues. The latter can be fatal if preventive measures are not undertaken.

What should you know about the drug?

Dilantin is useful for the control of grand mal seizures and psychomotor seizures. It is not effective against petit mal (absence) seizures.

Because the results of some studies suggest that this class of drug may cause birth defects in the developing fetus, its use during pregnancy is not advised.

Dilantin can interact with various other drugs. Some of these interactions can cause potentially serious complications. Consult your physician before taking any other drugs.

Are there any special precautions?

The use of Dilantin should be discontinued immediately at the first sign of a skin rash. Consult your physician if this occurs. The dosage may have to be reduced. If a rash occurs despite lowered dosage, further use of Dilantin is not advised.

Dimetane® Expectorant

Generic name

This product contains a combination of brompheniramine maleate, guaifenesin, phenylephrine hydrochloride, phenylpropanolamine hydrochloride, and alcohol.

Class of drug

Antihistamine, expectorant, and decongestant

In what form is the drug available?

Syrup

Why is the drug prescribed?

It is used to provide temporary relief from coughing and the complications of allergies such as hay fever (allergic rhinitis).

What are some possible side effects?

The most frequently encountered side effects include drowsiness, sedation, hives (urticaria) or drug-induced skin rash, chills, dryness of the mouth, nose and throat, sensitivity to light (photosensitivity), excessive perspiration, thickening of the secretions in the air passages (bronchial tubes), stuffy nose, and wheezing.

Some persons, while taking Dimetane Expectorant, have had a drop in blood pressure (hypotension), an abnormally rapid heartbeat (tachycardia), a sensation of the heartbeat (palpitations), and high blood pressure (hypertension). The drug may also cause extreme excitability (hysteria), retention of urine, and difficulty urinating.

More serious side effects occasionally occur. These include convulsions, severe allergic reactions (anaphylactic shock), and impairment of the blood-forming tissues.

What should you know about the drug?

The FDA, based partly on a review of this drug by the

National Academy of Sciences, states that Dimetane Expectorant is "lacking substantial evidence of effectiveness as a fixed combination for relief of coughing and for symptomatic relief of many manifestations of allergic states in which expectorant action is desired."

Are there any special precautions?

The manufacturer states that experience with the brompheniramine maleate ingredient of Dimetane Expectorant is insufficient in deciding whether or not it can cause harm to the developing fetus. This ingredient also exerts an additive effect when taken with alcohol, sedatives, tranquilizers, or other depressants of the central nervous system. Caution must be taken when driving, operating potentially dangerous machinery, or engaging in other activities where mental alertness is essential.

Dimetane Expectorant should not be taken by nursing mothers.

Overdose of this drug in infants and children may cause hallucinations, convulsions, or death.

Dimetapp®

Generic name

This product contains a combination of brompheniramine maleate, phenylephrine hydrochloride, phenylpropanolamine hydrochloride, and alcohol.

Class of drug

Antihistamine and decongestant

In what form is the drug available?

Elixir (liquid form to be taken by mouth) and tablets (Extentab®)

Why is the drug prescribed?

It is used to relieve the symptoms of hay fever (allergic rhinitis), nasal congestion, and runny nose.

What are some possible side effects?

The most frequently encountered side effects are drowsiness and a sensation of the heartbeat (palpitations). Because of the similarity of ingredients, other possible side effects are listed under Dimetane Expectorant.

What should you know about the drug?

This product contains the same ingredients as Dimetane Expectorant, with the exception of guaifenesin,
an expectorant which helps loosen secretions in the air
passages to aid in their expulsion by the cough reflex.

Are there any special precautions?

Precautions in the use of Dimetapp are virtually the
same as for Dimetane Expectorant.

Diupres®

Generic name

This product contains a combination of chlorothiazide
and reserpine.

Class of drug

Diuretic and antihypertensive

In what form is the drug available?

Tablets

Why is the drug prescribed?

It is used to treat patients with high blood pressure
(hypertension).

   The two ingredients in Diupres act together to lower
blood pressure (antihypertensive action) and eliminate
the accumulation of excessive amounts of water and
salt from the tissues (diuretic action).

What are some possible side effects?

The more frequently encountered side effects include
loss of appetite (anorexia), stomach irritation, nausea,
vomiting, cramps, diarrhea, constipation, dizziness,
headache, sedation, stuffy nose (nasal congestion), and
dryness of the mouth.

   Less frequently, other side effects may be experienced. These include: mental depression, blurred vision, a drop in blood pressure (hypotension), skin
rashes, sensitivity of the eyes to light (photosensitivity), drug-induced fever, muscle spasm, and jaundice.

   Some patients, while taking Diupres, occasionally
experience much more serious side effects. These include severe allergic reactions (anaphylactic shock)
and impairment of the blood-forming tissues.

What should you know about the drug?

Physicians have been warned that Diupres, a fixed combination drug, is not indicated for initial therapy in patients with hypertension. As with all potent drugs, the dosage of Diupres must be adjusted according to the response of the individual patient.

This drug is *not* for use in patients with known suicidal tendencies, active mental depression, peptic ulcer, or ulcerative colitis (an inflammatory disease of the large intestine). Diupres must be used with caution in patients with diabetes, gout, heart failure, severe kidney disease, and liver disease.

Are there any special precautions?

Diupres must be used with extreme caution (if at all) during pregnancy. The drug should *not* be used by nursing mothers.

Patients taking Diupres should have periodic tests to determine if the drug has adversely affected the body's normal balance of serum electrolytes (essential salts and other substances in the body tissues and fluids).

Oversedation may occur if Diupres is taken with alcohol, sedatives, tranquilizers, or other substances that depress the central nervous system.

Diuril®

Generic name
Chlorothiazide

Class of drug
Diuretic and antihypertensive

In what form is the drug available?
Tablets and oral suspension (liquid form to be taken by mouth)

Why is the drug prescribed?
It is used to eliminate the accumulation of excessive amounts of water and salt from the tissues (diuretic action) and to reduce high blood pressure (antihypertensive action). Water accumulation (edema) is one result of several disorders, including congestive heart failure, kidney disease, and cirrhosis of the liver.

Diuril can be used alone or in combination with

other drugs in the treatment of high blood pressure (hypertension).

What are some possible side effects?

The more frequently encountered side effects include loss of appetite (anorexia), stomach irritation, nausea, vomiting, cramps, diarrhea, constipation, dizziness, headache, and restlessness.

Side effects experienced less frequently include blurred vision, sensitivity of the eyes to light (photosensitivity), a drop in blood pressure (hypotension), skin rashes, drug-induced fever, muscle spasms, and jaundice.

Much more serious side effects occasionally occur in patients taking Diuril. These include a severe allergic reaction (anaphylactic shock) and impairment of the blood-forming tissues.

What should you know about the drug?

As with all potent drugs, the dosage of Diuril must be adjusted according to the response of the individual patient.

Diuril must be used with caution in patients with diabetes, gout, severe kidney disease, and liver disease.

Are there any special precautions?

Diuril must be used with extreme caution (if at all) during pregnancy. The drug should *not* be used by nursing mothers.

Patients taking Diuril should have periodic tests to determine if the drug has adversely affected the body's normal balance of serum electrolytes (essential salts and other substances in the body tissues and fluids).

Donnatal®

Generic name

This product contains a combination of phenobarbital, hyoscyamine sulfate, atropine sulfate, and hyoscine hydrobromide.

Class of drug

Anticholinergic (antispasmodic) and mild sedative

In what form is the drug available?

Tablets, capsules, and elixir (a liquid form to be taken by mouth)

Why is the drug prescribed?

It is used to treat the symptoms of various intestinal disorders and to relieve symptoms associated with peptic ulcers.

What are some possible side effects?

The most frequently encountered side effects include blurred vision, dry mouth, difficulty in urinating, and flushing or dryness of the skin. These side effects may occur in patients taking a high dosage of the drug but rarely in those taking the usual dosage.

What should you know about the drug?

The FDA, based partly on a review of Donnatal by the National Academy of Sciences, states that this drug is "possibly effective" as part of the therapy for the following conditions: peptic ulcer; the irritable bowel syndrome (irritable colon, spastic colon, mucous colitis); and acute enterocolitis.

Although the amount of phenobarbital in Donnatal is relatively small, this ingredient can be habit-forming.

Donnatal does not *cure* disease. It only relieves the cramps and spasms associated with certain disorders of the gastrointestinal system.

Are there any special precautions?

Donnatal should not be used in persons who are allergic to any of its ingredients.

This drug must be used with caution in patients with enlargement of the prostate gland, obstruction of the neck of the bladder, glaucoma, and chronic disease of the lungs.

Consult your physician before taking any other medication at the same time as Donnatal.

Doriden®

Generic name
Glutethimide

Class of drug
Hypnotic (sleeping pill) and sedative

In what form is the drug available?
Tablets

Why is the drug prescribed?
It is used to help induce sleep in persons with insomnia or poor sleeping habits.

What are some possible side effects?
The most frequently encountered side effects include nausea, morning hangover, blurred vision, and excitation. Some patients taking Doriden may also experience a generalized skin rash.

What should you know about the drug?
The sedative action of Doriden takes effect shortly after the drug is swallowed. Do not drive, operate potentially dangerous machinery, or engage in other tasks that demand mental alertness until the individual effects of the drug on a particular person are known. The sedative effects of Doriden are further increased, sometimes dangerously, by taking alcohol, tranquilizers, or other substances that depress the central nervous system.

Doriden can cause both psychological and physical dependence, especially with prolonged use.

If use of Doriden is abruptly discontinued it can produce severe withdrawal symptoms. These include: nausea, abdominal pain, tremors, delirium, and convulsions. Newborn babies of mothers who have taken Doriden for prolonged periods during their pregnancy may also suffer symptoms of drug withdrawal.

Are there any special precautions?
Doriden should *not* be used during pregnancy. Further, this drug should not be made available to persons with known suicidal tendencies.

Drixoral®

Generic name
This product contains a combination of dexbrompheniramine maleate and pseudoephedrine sulfate.

Class of drug
Antihistamine and decongestant

In what form is the drug available?
Tablets

Why is the drug prescribed?
It is used to relieve runny nose and stuffy nose (nasal congestion) associated with the common cold and allergies such as hay fever (allergic rhinitis).

Drixoral is also used in the treatment of blockage or congestion of the Eustachian tube, the canal that connects the middle ear to the upper part of the throat, and which acts to equalize the air pressure on each side of the eardrum.

What are some possible side effects?
The most frequently encountered side effects include drowsiness, mental confusion, restlessness, nausea, vomiting, drug-induced rashes, dizziness, loss of appetite (anorexia), a sensation of the heartbeat (palpitations), headache, insomnia, anxiety, an increase in the heartbeat (tachycardia), difficulty urinating, abdominal cramps, and sweating.

Some patients have also experienced a rise in blood pressure (hypertension) and shock.

What should you know about the drug?
The possible sedative effects of Drixoral can be increased by taking alcohol, sedatives, tranquilizers, or other substances that depress the central nervous system. Caution must be taken when driving or operating potentially dangerous machinery until the effects of the drug are known on an individual patient.

Consult your physician before taking any other drugs at the same time as Drixoral.

Are there any special precautions?
Drixoral should not be used during pregnancy or by nursing mothers. The safety of the drug during pregnancy and lactation has not yet been established.

Drixoral should not be given to children under the age of twelve. It should be used with caution in patients with high blood pressure, coronary artery disease, glaucoma, disease of the prostate gland, overactive thyroid gland (hyperthyroidism), and diabetes.

Dyazide®

Generic name
This product contains a combination of triamterene and hydrochlorothiazide.

Class of drug
Diuretic and antihypertensive

In what form is the drug available?
Capsules

Why is the drug prescribed?
It is used to eliminate the accumulation of excessive amounts of water and salt from the tissues (diuretic action). Water accumulation (edema) is one result of several disorders, including congestive heart failure, cirrhosis of the liver, and the nephrotic syndrome (a condition marked by high levels of protein in the urine, abnormally low levels of albumin in the blood, and excessive accumulation of water in the tissues).

The triamterene ingredient in this combination tends to curb the loss of the essential mineral potassium through the kidneys. This could occur if the hydrochlorothiazide component were prescribed alone.

Dyazide is also used in the treatment of high blood pressure (hypertension) when edema is an underlying problem.

What are some possible side effects?
The most frequently encountered side effects include muscle cramps, weakness, dizziness, headache, dry mouth, sensitivity to light (photosensitivity), nausea, vomiting, diarrhea, constipation, and drug-induced rash.

A few patients have experienced a severe allergic reaction (anaphylactic shock) while taking Dyazide.

What should you know about the drug?
Dyazide does not ordinarily flush out potassium through the kidneys. Because of this, there is a possible danger in some patients that excessive amounts of potassium will accumulate in the body. This is especially true if the patient is taking supplementary doses of this mineral. Blood tests at intervals during therapy will alert a physician to any dangerous increase in the body's level of potassium.

Are there any special precautions?

Dyazide should be used with extreme caution (if at all) during pregnancy. The drug should *not* be used by nursing mothers.

Elavil®

Generic name
Amitriptyline hydrochloride

Class of drug
Antidepressant

In what form is the drug available?
Tablets (an injectable form is also available)

Why is the drug prescribed?
It is used to relieve symptoms of depression. In persons who have experienced moderately severe depression and anxiety for some time, Elavil tends to improve mental alertness, elevate mood, and improve sleep.

What are some possible side effects?
The most frequently encountered side effects include drowsiness, dizziness, dry mouth, blurred vision, confusion, difficulty urinating, and constipation.

Some patients taking this class of drug occasionally experience high blood pressure (hypertension), a drop in blood pressure (hypotension), disturbances in the heart rhythm (cardiac arrhythmias), drug-induced rashes, and impairment of the blood-forming tissues.

What should you know about the drug?
Elavil falls within the general group of drugs known as tricyclic antidepressants. These drugs are not considered to be true tranquilizers and should not be prescribed on a casual basis. It usually takes from two to three weeks before their therapeutic effects are experienced.

Are there any special precautions?
Elavil should be used with extreme caution in patients with a particular form of glaucoma (narrow-angle glaucoma), retention of urine, a history of convulsive seizures, and in patients recovering from a recent heart attack.

Elavil must not be taken at the same time as drugs known as monoamine oxidase (MAO) inhibitors. Otherwise, extremely serious reactions may occur, including high fever, convulsions, and death. Elavil may also reduce the effectiveness of the antihypertensive drug Ismelin.

Alcohol, sedatives, tranquilizers, and other depressants of the central nervous system can cause oversedation if taken at the same time as Elavil. Use caution when driving, operating potentially dangerous machinery, or performing other tasks where mental alertness is essential, until the effects of the drug are known in a particular individual.

Elavil should be used with caution during pregnancy because its possible effect on the developing fetus has not yet been established.

Empirin® Compound with Codeine

Generic name
This product contains a combination of aspirin, phenacetin, caffeine, and codeine phosphate.

Class of drug
Combination of narcotic analgesic and nonnarcotics

In what form is the drug available?
Tablets

Why is the drug prescribed?
It is used as an analgesic (pain reliever).

What are some possible side effects?
As with all combination products, the possible side effects are those associated with the individual ingredients. People who are sensitive to aspirin may experience stomach irritation, pain, and nausea. In some cases aspirin, especially in large quantities, may cause bleeding of the stomach lining.

The phenacetin ingredient can cause kidney damage in a few individuals, especially if taken in large doses continually over a period of months.

The codeine ingredient is a narcotic drug. It can cause drowsiness, nausea, and constipation. As with any narcotic, extended use of codeine is accompanied by the risk of addiction. Excessive use of codeine carries the risk of extremely serious side effects including, in cases of severe overdose, shock, cardiac arrest (stopping of the heart), and death.

The caffeine ingredient is a mild stimulant. Overdose can cause insomnia, restlessness, excitement, and an increase in the heart rate (tachycardia).

The most frequently encountered side effects associated with the use of Empirin Compound with Codeine include lightheadedness, dizziness, sedation, nausea, and vomiting.

What should you know about the drug?

The sedative effect of the codeine ingredient in this product can be increased by taking alcohol, tranquilizers, or other substances that depress the central nervous system. Use caution when driving, operating potentially dangerous machinery, or engaging in tasks that require mental alertness.

Are there any special precautions?

Empirin Compound with Codeine should be used with caution (if at all) during pregnancy. Consult your physician before taking any other drugs at the same time as Empirin Compound with Codeine.

Enduron®

Generic name
Methyclothiazide

Class of drug
Diuretic and antihypertensive

In what form is the drug available?
Tablets

Why is the drug prescribed?

It is used to eliminate the accumulation of excessive amounts of water and salt from the tissues (diuretic action) and to reduce high blood pressure (antihypertensive action). Water accumulation (edema) is one result of several disorders, including congestive heart failure and cirrhosis of the liver. Edema can also occur as a consequence of corticosteroid and estrogen therapy.

Enduron is also used to treat various forms of kidney disease when edema is a problem.

What are some possible side effects?

The most frequently encountered side effects include loss of appetite (anorexia), stomach irritation, nausea, vomiting, cramps, muscle spasm, diarrhea, constipation, dizziness, headache, sensitivity of the eyes to light (photosensitivity), and drug-induced rashes.

Some patients, while taking Enduron, have also experienced the following: jaundice; hypersensitivity (allergic) reactions; a drop in blood pressure which may be made worse by taking alcohol, sedatives, or narcotic drugs; and impairment of the blood-forming tissues.

What should you know about the drug?

Enduron may cause a loss of potassium by the kidneys. Blood tests at intervals during therapy will indicate such an imbalance and can be treated with potassium supplements.

Are there any special precautions?

Enduron should be used with extreme caution (if at all) during pregnancy. The drug should *not* be used by nursing mothers.

Equagesic®

Generic name

This product contains a combination of meprobamate, ethoheptazine citrate, and aspirin.

Class of drug

Analgesic

In what form is the drug available?

Tablets

Why is the drug prescribed?

It is used to relieve pain associated with tension or anxiety in patients with disease of the muscles, bones, and joints (musculoskeletal disease), or headache.

What are some possible side effects?

The most frequently encountered side effects are nausea, vomiting, and abdominal pain or discomfort.

Drowsiness may occur in some patients, but usually disappears with continued therapy.

Some patients have had drug-induced skin rashes. Physical and psychological dependence to meprobamate can occur with chronic use.

The aspirin ingredient of this product may cause bleeding of the stomach lining in some individuals.

What should you know about the drug?

The FDA, based partly on a review of this drug by the National Academy of Sciences, states that Equagesic is "possibly effective" in the treatment of pain accompanied by tension or anxiety in patients with musculoskeletal disease or tension headache.

The manufacturer has cautioned that physicians should periodically reassess the usefulness of Equagesic for the individual patient.

Are there any special precautions?

Equagesic should not be used during pregnancy. The drug should not be used by nursing mothers. There is a risk of damage to the developing fetus with the use of minor tranquilizers, such as meprobamate (an ingredient of Equagesic). Meprobamate is present in breast milk of mothers who take this drug.

Equagesic should not be given to children twelve years of age and under.

erythromycin

Brand names

Bristamycin® E.E.S.® E-Mycin® Erythrocin® Ethril® Ilosone® Ilotycin® Pediamycin® Pfizer-E® Robimycin® SK-Erythromycin® Wyamycin®

Class of drug

Antibiotic

In what form is the drug available?

Erythromycin is available in several different chemical compositions and various dosage forms depending on the manufacturer. These include: tablets, chewable tablets, capsules, oral suspension, pediatric suspension, pediatric drops, suppositories, skin ointment, and eye ointment.

Why is the drug prescribed?

It is used mainly to treat relatively mild or moderate bacterial infections, especially when the bacteria are resistant to the effects of penicillin. Erythromycin is also often prescribed when the patient is allergic to penicillin.

Erythromycin is not the drug of first choice to treat severe bacterial infections. It tends to inhibit the growth and multiplication of bacteria (bacteriostatic action), rather than destroy them (bactericidal action).

What are some possible side effects?

According to the American Medical Association in its publication *AMA Drug Evaluations,* erythromycin "is considered to be one of the safer antibiotics in use today." With the exception of one form of the drug (erythromycin estolate, available as Ilosone), serious adverse reactions are rarely encountered.

What should you know about the drug?

One form of erythromycin (Ilosone) should not be taken by patients with a known history of liver disease or impaired liver function. This form has been known to cause liver damage and jaundice.

As with all antibiotics, erythromycin should be taken exactly as prescribed by your physician. Do not stop taking the drug just because you feel better. Complete the full course of therapy as directed on the label.

Are there any special precautions?

Overdose with erythromycin may cause abdominal discomfort, diarrhea, nausea, and vomiting.

Prolonged use of any antibiotic may result in the development of infections by other species of microorganisms (bacteria and fungi).

Liquid forms of erythromycin should be kept in a refrigerator and not used if they are over fourteen days old.

Fiorinal®

Generic name

This product contains a combination of butalbital, aspirin, phenacetin, and caffeine.

Class of drug
Analgesic

In what form is the drug available?
Tablets and capsules

Why is the drug prescribed?
It is used to relieve pain, especially in the treatment of tension headache (headache pain, mental tension, and muscle contraction in the head, neck, and shoulders).

What are some possible side effects?
The most frequently encountered side effects are drowsiness and dizziness. Less frequent side effects include lightheadedness, nausea, vomiting, flatulence, and other disturbances of the digestive system.

The aspirin ingredient of this product may cause bleeding of the stomach lining in some individuals.

More serious side effects, attributable to the individual ingredients, have been reported in cases of overdose.

What should you know about the drug?
The butalbital ingredient of Fiorinal can be habit-forming, especially if taken for prolonged periods. The sedative effect of the drug can be increased if taken with alcohol, tranquilizers, or other substances that depress the central nervous system. Use caution when driving, operating potentially dangerous machinery, or performing tasks that require mental alertness until the effects of the drug are known on an individual patient.

Are there any special precautions?
Because Fiorinal contains aspirin it should be used with extreme caution by patients with peptic ulcer or blood-clotting abnormalities. Consult your physician if you are taking any other drugs at the same time, especially those prescribed to thin the blood.

The phenacetin ingredient can cause kidney damage in a few individuals, especially if taken continually over a period of months.

Fiorinal® with Codeine

Generic name
This product contains a combination of codeine phosphate, butalbital, aspirin, phenacetin, and caffeine.

Class of drug
Narcotic analgesic

In what form is the drug available?
Capsules

Why is the drug prescribed?
It is used to relieve moderate to severe pain in a variety of conditions, especially those in which the more potent painkilling (analgesic) effect of morphine is not required.

What are some possible side effects?
The most frequently encountered side effects include nausea, vomiting, constipation, drug-induced skin rashes, drowsiness, and contraction of the pupils of the eyes (miosis).

What should you know about the drug?
With the exception of codeine phosphate (a narcotic analgesic), this product contains the same ingredients as Fiorinal (see above).

The codeine phosphate and butalbital ingredients of this product can be habit-forming, especially if taken for prolonged periods. The sedative effects of the drug can be increased if taken with alcohol, tranquilizers, or other substances that depress the central nervous system. Use caution when driving, operating potentially dangerous machinery, or performing tasks that require mental alertness.

Are there any special precautions?
Codeine or any drug containing codeine can be addictive. Overdosage can lead to serious complications. Take Fiorinal with Codeine exactly as prescribed by your physician. Report any adverse effects at once.

Other precautions in the use of this drug are exactly the same as those listed for Fiorinal.

Flagyl®

Generic name
Metronidazole

Class of drug
Antiprotozoal/amebicide

In what form is the drug available?
Tablets

Why is the drug prescribed?
It is used primarily in the treatment of a condition known as trichomoniasis, an infection with protozoal microorganisms of the species *Trichomonas vaginalis*. In women this disorder causes inflammation of the vagina (vaginitis). The infection is usually acquired during sexual intercourse.

In addition to vaginitis, it may cause inflammation of the bladder (cystitis) and the passage from the bladder through which urine passes (urethritis). Men are affected less commonly than women, but may be carriers of the disease.

Flagyl is also used in the treatment of acute intestinal amebiasis (amebic dysentery) and amebic liver abscess.

What are some possible side effects?
The most frequently encountered side effects include nausea, loss of appetite (anorexia), and a metallic taste.

Less frequently the side effects include headache, dizziness, and a burning sensation while urinating. Serious side effects are unusual.

What should you know about the drug?
Flagyl is especially effective against protozoa (single-celled organisms) of the species *Trichomonas vaginalis* (which cause trichomoniasis), and *Entamoeba histolytica* (which cause amebic dysentery).

The manufacturer warns that in experimental studies, Flagyl has been shown to cause cancer in mice and possibly in rats. Thus, Flagyl should not be used casually, but should be restricted to the specific conditions outlined above. There is no evidence that the drug can cause cancer in humans, but the possibility exists nevertheless.

In some patients, a drug interaction occurs if alcohol is taken at the same time as Flagyl. This can cause nausea, vomiting, headaches, faintness, and flushing.

Are there any special precautions?

Flagyl should *not* be used during the first three months of pregnancy. It should be used with extreme caution (if at all) throughout the later stages of pregnancy. The drug should not be taken by nursing mothers.

Flagyl should not be used in persons with blood disorders or in those with active disease of the central nervous system.

Gantanol®

Generic name
Sulfamethoxazole

Class of drug
Antibacterial (sulfonamide)

In what form is the drug available?
Tablets and oral suspension

Why is the drug prescribed?
It is used to treat infections of the urinary tract.

What are some possible side effects?
The most frequently encountered side effects are nausea, vomiting, headache, and dizziness. Some patients taking Gantanol (a sulfa drug) may experience allergic reactions, including skin rashes. Life-threatening allergic reactions (anaphylactic shock) also have occurred in patients taking this class of drug, in addition to severe impairment of the blood-forming tissues.

What should you know about the drug?
Gantanol should be used with caution in patients with impaired function of the kidneys or liver, bronchial asthma, or severe allergies.

Gantanol must *not* be used in the treatment of strep throat (streptococcal pharyngitis).

Are there any special precautions?
Drink plenty of water or other fluids while being

treated with Gantanol. This helps prevent the formation of crystals of the drug, which could lodge in the kidneys and cause serious damage.

Discontinue the use of Gantanol and consult your physician immediately at the first sign of skin rashes, sore throat, pallor, or yellowness of the skin (a sign of jaundice). Gantanol should not be used during pregnancy or during the nursing period. Consult your physician before taking any other drugs at the same time as Gantanol.

Gantrisin®

Generic name
Sulfisoxazole

Class of drug
Antibacterial (sulfonamide)

In what form is the drug available?
Tablets, pediatric suspension and syrup, and injectable

Why is the drug prescribed?
It is used mainly to treat bacterial infections of the urinary tract, including infections of the bladder (cystitis) and kidney (pyelitis and pyelonephritis).

What are some possible side effects?
The most frequently encountered side effects include nausea, vomiting, abdominal pain, diarrhea, headache, dizziness, mental depression, a ringing in the ears (tinnitus), and insomnia.

Less frequently encountered side effects include hallucinations, drug-induced fever, chills, and, with the injectable form of Gantrisin, inflammation at the site of injection.

As is true with other sulfa drugs, some patients have experienced more serious side effects. These include: kidney damage, convulsions, severe allergic reactions (anaphylactic shock), and impairment of the blood-forming tissues.

What should you know about the drug?
Physicians have been advised by the manufacturer to use the injectable form of Gantrisin only when administration by mouth is impractical for any reason.

It is essential to take this drug exactly as instructed by the physician. Complete the full course of therapy, even if you feel better.

Are there any special precautions?

Gantrisin should not be used during pregnancy or if the mother is nursing.

Gantrisin should be used with extreme caution (if at all) in persons with kidney disease, liver disease, bronchial asthma, and severe allergies.

It is important to drink plenty of water or other fluids while taking Gantrisin. This helps minimize the risk of kidney stones (the formation of crystals of the drug).

Consult your physician at the first sign of fever, jaundice, sore throat, or other possible side effects associated with the use of Gantrisin.

Hydergine®

Generic name

This product contains a combination of three dihydro derivatives of ergot alkaloids.

Class of drug

Psychotherapeutic

In what form is the drug available?

Tablets and sublingual tablets (dissolved under the tongue)

Why is the drug prescribed?

The manufacturer claims that Hydergine can have some benefit for the elderly in relieving confusion, depression, dizziness, and antisocial behavior.

What are some possible side effects?

The most frequently encountered side effects include nausea, disturbances of the digestive tract, blurred vision, stuffy nose, and skin rashes. However, the manufacturer claims that Hydergine has not been found to produce any serious adverse effects.

What should you know about the drug?

The American Medical Association, in their publication *AMA Drug Evaluations,* states: "There is no convincing evidence that Hydergine is useful in patients with severe mental impairment, except possibly in those with organic brain syndrome due to hypertension."

Are there any special precautions?
Overdosage with Hydergine may impair the blood flow to the arms and legs. Take this drug exactly as prescribed by your physician.

hydrochlorothiazide

Brand names
Esidrix® HydroDIURIL® Oretic®

Class of drug
Diuretic and antihypertensive

In what form is the drug available?
Tablets

Why is the drug prescribed?
It helps the kidneys flush out excessive amounts of water and salt from the tissues. Water retention causes swelling of the tissues (edema) and is one result of several disorders. These include congestive heart failure, cirrhosis of the liver, and various forms of kidney disease. Edema can also occur as a consequence of corticosteroid and estrogen therapy.

Used either alone or in combination with other drugs, hydrochlorothiazide is used to help lower blood pressure in cases of hypertension.

What are some possible side effects?
The most frequently encountered side effects include loss of appetite (anorexia), stomach irritation, nausea, vomiting, cramps, diarrhea, constipation, dizziness, headache, increased sensitivity of the eyes to light (photosensitivity), drug-induced rashes, weakness, restlessness, and blurred vision.

Less frequently encountered side effects include fever, jaundice, and a drop in blood pressure (hypotension).

A few patients receiving hydrochlorothiazide have experienced severe allergic reactions (anaphylactic shock) and impairment of the blood-forming tissues.

What should you know about the drug?

The use of hydrochlorothiazide may cause an excessive loss of the essential mineral potassium through the kidneys. This is especially possible if the drug is taken at higher doses or used for prolonged periods. The side effects that occur with diminished levels of potassium in the body can be minimized or avoided by eating foods rich in potassium such as fruit juice, dried fruits, and bananas. The physician may also prescribe potassium supplements.

Are there any special precautions?

Hydrochlorothiazide should be used with extreme caution (if at all) during pregnancy. It should *not* be used to treat uncomplicated edema often experienced by pregnant women. Routine use of diuretics (water pills) exposes both mother and fetus to unnecessary risks.

This drug should be used with caution in patients with disease of the kidneys or liver.

Consult your physician before taking any other drugs at the same time as hydrochlorothiazide.

Hydropres®

Generic name
This product contains a combination of hydrochlorothiazide and reserpine.

Class of drug
Diuretic and antihypertensive

In what form is the drug available?
Tablets

Why is the drug prescribed?
It is used to treat patients with high blood pressure (hypertension).

The two ingredients in Hydropres act together to lower blood pressure (antihypertensive action) and eliminate the accumulation of excessive amounts of water and salt from the tissues (diuretic action).

What are some possible side effects?
The more frequently encountered side effects include loss of appetite (anorexia), stomach irritation, nausea, vomiting, cramps, diarrhea, constipation, dizziness,

headache, stuffy nose (nasal congestion), sedation, and dryness of the mouth.

Less frequently encountered side effects include blurred vision, a drop in blood pressure (hypotension), skin rashes, sensitivity of the eyes to light (photosensitivity), drug-induced fever, muscle spasm, and jaundice.

In a few cases, patients taking this combination product have experienced more serious side effects. These include severe allergic reactions (anaphylactic shock) and impairment of the blood-forming tissues.

What should you know about the drug?

Physicians have been warned by the FDA, based on a report from the National Academy of Sciences, that Hydropres, a fixed combination drug, "is not indicated for initial therapy of hypertension." As with all potent drugs, the dosage of Hydropres must be adjusted according to the response of the individual.

This drug is *not* for use in patients with known suicidal tendencies, active mental depression, peptic ulcer, or ulcerative colitis (an inflammatory disease of the large intestine). Hydropres must be used with caution in patients with diabetes, gout, heart failure, severe kidney disease, and liver disease.

Patients taking Hydropres should have periodic tests to determine if the drug has adversely affected the body's normal balance of serum electrolytes (essential salts and other substances in the body tissues and fluids).

Are there any special precautions?

Hydropres must be used with extreme caution (if at all) during pregnancy. The drug should *not* be used by nursing mothers.

Oversedation may occur if Hydropres is taken with alcohol, sedatives, tranquilizers, or other substances that depress the central nervous system.

Hygroton®

Generic name
Chlorthalidone

Class of drug
Diuretic and antihypertensive

In what form is the drug available?

Tablets

Why is the drug prescribed?

Hygroton often is used with other drugs to eliminate the accumulation of excessive amounts of water and salt from the tissues (diuretic action) and to lower blood pressure (antihypertensive action).

The accumulation of water in the tissues causes them to swell (edema). Edema is one result of several disorders, including congestive heart failure and cirrhosis of the liver, and as a consequence of corticosteroid and estrogen therapy.

What are some possible side effects?

The most frequently encountered side effects include loss of appetite (anorexia), stomach irritation, nausea, vomiting, cramps, diarrhea, constipation, and restlessness.

Some patients taking Hygroton may experience other side effects, including drug-induced skin rashes, jaundice, the inability to achieve or maintain an erection of the penis (impotence), and impairment of the blood-forming tissues.

What should you know about the drug?

Hygroton has a prolonged action: its therapeutic effects last approximately forty-eight to seventy-two hours.

Individuals with a history of allergies or bronchial asthma may occasionally experience a sensitivity (allergic) reaction while taking Hygroton.

This drug should be used with caution in patients with disease of the kidneys or liver.

Patients taking Hygroton should have periodic tests to determine if the drug has adversely affected the body's normal balance of serum electrolytes (essential salts and other substances in the body tissues and fluids).

Are there any special precautions?

Hygroton should be used with extreme caution (if at all) during pregnancy. It should *not* be used by nursing mothers.

Inderal®

Generic name
Propranolol hydrochloride

Class of drug
Beta-adrenergic blocking agent/antihypertensive

In what form is the drug available?
Tablets (an injectable form is also available)

Why is the drug prescribed?
It is used mainly to treat high blood pressure (hypertension), angina pectoris (chest pains caused by a temporarily insufficient supply of blood to the heart muscle), and specific types of irregular or abnormal heart rhythms.

What are some possible side effects?
The most frequently encountered side effects include tiredness, mental depression, lightheadedness, visual disturbances, a reduced heart rate (bradycardia), temporary loss of memory, excitability, and mental confusion. These side effects tend to occur during the early period of therapy.

More severe side effects have been reported in a few patients taking Inderal. These include: congestive heart failure, a drop in blood pressure (hypotension), impairment of the blood-forming tissues, aggravation of diabetes, and arterial insufficiency in the extremities in those with Raynaud's disease.

What should you know about the drug?
The effects of Inderal in controlling high blood pressure are enhanced if therapy includes the use of a diuretic (water pill) such as hydrochlorothiazide.

The dosage of Inderal must be carefully adjusted to the needs of the individual patient for maximum effect. This may require several weeks to achieve. Inderal may precipitate asthmatic attacks in susceptible patients.

If Inderal therapy is suddenly stopped it may cause serious complications. These include the recurrence of attacks of angina pectoris (chest pains), an increase in the heart rate (tachycardia), heart attack (myocardial infarction), and sudden death. To avert or minimize these risks, the dosage of Inderal must be gradually reduced over a period of one or two weeks before the drug is discontinued.

Are there any special precautions?

It is essential to take Inderal exactly as prescribed by your physician. Extremely serious consequences can occur in some people if use of the drug is suddenly stopped.

The safe use of Inderal during pregnancy has not been established.

Indocin®

Generic name
Indomethacin

Class of drug
Anti-inflammatory

In what form is the drug available?
Capsules

Why is the drug prescribed?

It is used to provide symptomatic relief of pain and disability associated with a wide variety of inflammation of the joints. These include: rheumatoid arthritis, ankylosing spondylitis (a progressive inflammatory disease of the spine), osteoarthritis of large joints (hips, knees, and shoulders), and gout (acute gouty arthritis).

What are some possible side effects?

The manufacturer of Indocin is one of the few to publish the side effects that have occurred during use of this drug according to the *percentage* of patients treated (based on 33 separate studies involving over 1,000 patients). The following side effects can be expected to occur: headache (over 10% of patients); nausea, with or without vomiting (from 3–9%); dyspepsia, including indigestion, heartburn, and abdominal discomfort (from 3–9%); and dizziness (from 3–9%).

The following side effects can be expected in less than 1% of patients who take Indocin: stomach bleeding, peptic ulcer, high blood pressure (hypertension), anxiety, convulsions, mental confusion, blurred vision, hearing disturbances (including deafness), chest pain, rapid fall in blood pressure, edema (swelling or puffiness of the tissues caused by fluid retention), hepatitis, jaundice, skin rashes, vaginal bleeding, and impairment of the blood-forming tissues.

What should you know about the drug?

Physicians have been cautioned that Indocin is an extremely potent drug and should not be considered a simple analgesic (painkiller). It should not be used casually.

Indocin should always be prescribed in the lowest possible effective dose and taken immediately after meals to minimize the risk of stomach irritation.

This drug is not ordinarily recommended for use in children fourteen years of age and under. Its safety in this group has not been established.

A few deaths, caused by perforation and uncontrolled bleeding of the digestive tract, have occurred in patients taking Indocin.

Greater care should be taken with elderly patients as they tend to experience more adverse reactions.

Are there any special precautions?

Indocin should not be used during pregnancy or by nursing mothers.

Indocin should be used with caution in patients with blood-clotting abnormalities.

Ionamin®

Generic name
Phentermine resin

Class of drug
Anorectic (appetite suppressant)

In what form is the drug available?
Capsules

Why is the drug prescribed?
It is used as an aid in the initial treatment of obese (overweight) persons to suppress appetite.

What are some possible side effects?
The most frequently encountered side effects include

nervousness, anxiety, dry mouth, headache, dizziness, diarrhea, constipation, increased heart rate (tachycardia), sensation of the heartbeat (palpitations), and a rise in blood pressure (hypertension).

Some patients taking Ionamin also experience skin rashes, an inability to achieve or maintain erection of the penis (impotence), and various mental changes, some of which resemble schizophrenia (associated mainly with drug overdose).

What should you know about the drug?

Ionamin (or any other appetite suppressant) should not be taken for prolonged periods. The ability of the drug to suppress appetite tends to lessen with continued use. In addition, psychological dependence on the drug often develops.

Many physicians and experts in nutrition consider the use of appetite-suppressant drugs a basically ineffective way to control weight problems. Dietary changes are essential.

Are there any special precautions?

Ionamin may impair the ability to drive, operate potentially dangerous machinery, or engage in other activities where mental alertness is essential.

Ionamin should not be used by people with heart disorders, irregular heart rhythms, or high blood pressure.

Consult your physician before taking any other drugs at the same time as Ionamin.

Isopto-Carpine®

Generic name
Pilocarpine hydrochloride

Class of drug
Antiglaucomatous agent

In what form is the drug available?
Eyedrops

Why is the drug prescribed?
It is used in the treatment of glaucoma, a disease in which an abnormally high fluid pressure builds up within the eyeball. Isopto-Carpine causes a fall in

pressure within the eyeball. This reduces the risk of permanent loss of vision that could result from pressure damage to the optic nerve.

What are some possible side effects?
Local irritation, allergic reactions, and other adverse effects are uncommon when Isopto-Carpine is used exactly as prescribed.

What should you know about the drug?
Isopto-Carpine exerts its effect by causing the pupil to constrict. This typically occurs within fifteen to thirty minutes and lasts from four to eight hours.

In addition to lowering the pressure within the eye, Isopto-Carpine may also inhibit the production of more fluid (aqueous humor) within the eye.

Are there any special precautions?
When applying the solution, do not contaminate the eyedropper by touching the eye.

Isordil®

Generic name
Isosorbide dinitrate

Class of drug
Antianginal agent

In what form is the drug available?
Chewable tablets, sublingual tablets (a form which dissolves and is absorbed when placed under the tongue), sustained-action tablets and capsules (formulated for gradual release of the drug in the body over a period of about six hours), and Titradose E.Z. Split tablets for easy dosage adjustment)

Why is the drug prescribed?
It is used in the treatment of patients with angina pectoris to decrease the frequency and severity of chest pain. The pain is the result of a temporarily insufficient supply of blood to the heart muscle through the coronary arteries.

What are some possible side effects?
The most frequently encountered side effects are flush-

ing, headache, temporary bouts of dizziness and weakness, and occasionally, drug-induced skin rashes.

A few patients taking Isordil may experience nausea, vomiting, weakness, pallor, a drop in blood pressure (hypotension), and collapse. Alcohol can intensify these effects.

What should you know about the drug?

The FDA, based partly on a review of this drug by the National Academy of Sciences, states that Isordil—in the form of chewable tablets and sublingual tablets—is "probably" effective for the treatment of acute anginal attacks and for their prevention "in situations likely to provoke such attacks."

The FDA considers Isordil "possibly" effective in the form of scored tablets and sustained-action tablets and capsules in controlling angina pectoris. These dosage forms are used for the prevention of angina pectoris. They are not intended to treat an acute attack once it has started.

Isordil is also available in a tablet form combined with phenobarbital. For information on additional side effects and precautions, see phenobarbital.

Are there any special precautions?

Notify your physician immediately if the prescribed dose of Isordil does not relieve anginal pain. He may decide to prescribe a different drug or increase the dosage of Isordil. Do not increase the prescribed dose without medical advice.

Keflex®

Generic name
Cephalexin

Class of drug
Antibiotic (cephalosporin)

In what form is the drug available?
Tablets, capsules, oral suspension, and pediatric drops

Why is the drug prescribed?
The manufacturer claims that Keflex is useful in the treatment of specific bacterial infections of the respiratory tract, middle ear (otitis media), the skin and soft

tissues, some bone infections, and urinary tract infections. However, penicillin is usually the drug of choice in the treatment of streptococcal infections, and as a preventive measure for rheumatic fever.

Good reasons for prescribing Keflex include those cases where a particular patient is allergic to a more effective antibiotic such as ampicillin, or where a specific bacterial infection is known to be especially sensitive to the effects of Keflex.

What are some possible side effects?

The most frequently encountered side effects include diarrhea, dizziness, vomiting, stomach upset, abdominal pain, and skin rashes.

Some patients taking Keflex have experienced headache, itching (particularly around the genitals and anus), inflammation of the vagina (vaginitis), and vaginal discharge.

Keflex is occasionally the cause of severe allergic reactions (anaphylactic shock).

What should you know about the drug?

Keflex is much more expensive than other antibiotics which are often more effective in treating a specific bacterial infection. The American Medical Association, in its publication *AMA Drug Evaluations,* has stated that Keflex "is not usually a drug of choice for systemic infections."

Patients who are allergic to penicillin may also be allergic to Keflex. Such patients should be tested for possible allergic reaction prior to administration of the drug and be closely monitored while on the drug.

The long-term use of Keflex, as well as other antibiotics, may result in overgrowth in the body of various species of microorganisms.

Are there any special precautions?

Keflex should be used with caution during pregnancy and during the nursing period.

Consult your physician before taking any other drugs at the same time as Keflex.

Kenalog®

Generic name
Triamcinolone acetonide

Class of drug
Synthetic corticosteroid (anti-inflammatory)

In what form is the drug available?
Cream, lotion, ointment, and spray

Why is the drug prescribed?
It is used topically (on the skin surface) to treat various inflammatory skin disorders.

What are some possible side effects?
The most frequently encountered side effects that result from the use of topical corticosteroids including Kenalog are itching, dry skin, a burning sensation, and skin eruptions. These occur at the site where the drug is applied, and are more common when a tight dressing is placed over the affected area of skin.

If Kenalog is applied to a wide area of the body for prolonged periods, the drug may be absorbed through the skin and cause additional problems.

What should you know about the drug?
If Kenalog causes local irritation of the skin, its use should be discontinued.

Skin infections do not respond to Kenalog. In such cases an appropriate antibacterial or antifungal agent should first be used to clear the infection. Applying Kenalog may cause the infection to spread.

Are there any special precautions?
Use Kenalog only under the close supervision of your physician. Do not apply the drug to areas of the skin that seem infected.

The safe use of Kenalog during pregnancy has not been established.

Kwell®

Generic name
Gamma benzene hexachloride

Class of drug
Parasiticide

In what form is the drug available?
Cream, lotion, and shampoo

Why is the drug prescribed?

It is used to destroy the following skin parasites: *Sarcoptes scabiei* (scabies), *Pediculus capitis* (head lice), and *Phthirus pubis* (crab lice) and their eggs.

What are some possible side effects?

In some persons, Kwell can cause skin eruptions at the site of application as the result of local irritation or an allergic reaction. Many patients experience persistent itching after treatment has been completed.

If ingested or left on the skin for prolonged periods, Kwell may cause more serious side effects, including those that involve the liver and blood cells.

What should you know about the drug?

The shampoo form of Kwell is effective only against head lice and crab lice. It should *not* be used as an ordinary shampoo or left on the head for prolonged periods. Routine use can increase the risk of local irritation.

If Kwell is ingested, call your physician immediately. And if Kwell comes in contact with the eyes, flush them out immediately with water.

Are there any special precautions?

Keep this product out of reach of infants and small children. Kwell is a poison if taken by mouth.

Lasix®

Generic name
Furosemide

Class of drug
Diuretic and antihypertensive

In what form is the drug available?
Tablets and oral solution (an injectable form is also available)

Why is the drug prescribed?
The retention of fluids causes swelling of the tissues (edema). This is one result of several disorders, including congestive heart failure, cirrhosis of the liver, and certain forms of kidney disease.

Lasix is used to eliminate the accumulation of excessive amounts of water and salt from the tissues (diuretic action) and to lower blood pressure (antihypertensive action). Lasix may be used for these purposes alone or in combination with other diuretic and antihypertensive drugs.

What are some possible side effects?

The most frequently encountered side effects include loss of appetite (anorexia), irritation of the mouth, stomach irritation, nausea, vomiting, cramps, diarrhea, constipation, dizziness, headache, blurred vision, a ringing in the ears (tinnitus), and impaired hearing.

Some patients also experience sensitivity of the eyes to light (photosensitivity), skin rashes, itching, muscle spasm, weakness, jaundice, and spasm of the urinary bladder.

Rarely, Lasix is responsible for causing impairment of the blood-forming tissues.

What should you know about the drug?

Lasix exerts a greater diuretic effect on the kidneys than many other drugs in its general class. Unless precaution is taken, serious depletion of the essential mineral potassium may occur. This risk is minimized by giving potassium supplements and eating foods rich in potassium such as dried fruit, bananas, or fruit juice.

Patients taking Lasix should have periodic tests to determine if the drug has adversely affected the body's normal balance of serum electrolytes (essential salts and other substances in the body tissues and fluids).

Consult your physician before taking any other drugs at the same time as Lasix.

Are there any special precautions?

The results of experimental studies with Lasix in animals show that this drug may cause fetal abnormalities. Lasix should not be taken during pregnancy or by nursing mothers.

Librax®

Generic name

This product contains a combination of chlordiazepoxide hydrochloride and clidinium bromide.

Class of drug

Minor tranquilizer and anticholinergic (antispasmodic)

In what form is the drug available?

Capsules

Why is the drug prescribed?

It is used in the treatment of peptic ulcer, the irritable bowel syndrome (irritable colon, spastic colon, mucous colitis), and acute enterocolitis (inflammation of the moist lining of the small and large intestines).

What are some possible side effects?

The most frequently encountered side effects include drowsiness, dizziness, mental confusion, dry mouth, blurred vision, impaired muscular coordination, skin rashes, swelling of the tissues caused by fluid retention (edema), menstrual irregularities, nausea, constipation, difficulty urinating, and an increase or decrease in sex drive (libido).

A few patients taking Librax have experienced jaundice, liver disorders, and impairment of the blood-forming tissues.

What should you know about the drug?

The clidinium bromide ingredient in Librax acts to decrease the frequency and severity of painful spasms or contractions of the stomach and intestines (antispasmodic action). The chlordiazepoxide hydrochloride ingredient tends to relieve any associated anxiety.

The FDA, based partly on a review of the drug by the National Academy of Sciences, states that Librax is "possibly" effective as supportive therapy in the conditions listed above.

Are there any special precautions?

If the administration of Librax is suddenly discontinued, the patient may experience anxiety, nightmares, and insomnia.

Librax may impair mental alertness. Use caution when driving, operating potentially dangerous machinery, or engaging in other activities where mental alertness is essential.

Librax should *not* be used during pregnancy. Evidence exists that the use of the tranquilizing ingredient chlordiazepoxide hydrochloride carries the risk of malformations of the developing fetus.

Librium®

Generic name
Chlordiazepoxide hydrochloride

Class of drug
Minor tranquilizer

In what form is the drug available?
Capsules and tablets (an injectable form is also available)

Why is the drug prescribed?
It is used to relieve anxiety and tension and to relieve the withdrawal symptoms in patients with acute alcoholism.

What are some possible side effects?
The most frequently encountered side effects include drowsiness, impaired muscular coordination (ataxia), mental confusion, skin eruptions, edema, menstrual irregularities, nausea, constipation, and an increase or decrease in sex drive (libido).

A few patients taking Librium have experienced jaundice, liver disorders, and impairment of the blood-forming tissues.

What should you know about the drug?
Prolonged use of Librium, especially in large doses, may cause psychological and physical dependence.

The American Medical Association, in its publication *AMA Drug Evaluations*, states that this drug "has a wide margin of safety and is essentially ineffective as a suicide agent."

The sedative effects of Librium can be increased by taking alcohol, antihistamines, barbiturates (sleeping pills), and narcotic drugs. Use caution when driving, operating potentially dangerous machinery, or engaging in other activities that require mental alertness.

Are there any special precautions?
Librium should *not* be used during pregnancy. Evidence exists that use of drugs in this class carries the risk of malformations of the developing fetus.

Lidex®

Generic name
Fluocinonide

Class of drug
Synthetic corticosteroid (anti-inflammatory)

In what form is the drug available?
Cream and ointment

Why is the drug prescribed?
It is used topically (on the skin surface) to treat various inflammatory skin disorders.

What are some possible side effects?
The most frequently encountered side effects that result from the use of topical corticosteroids such as Lidex are itching, dry skin, a burning sensation, and skin eruptions. These occur at the site where the drug is applied, and are more common when a tight dressing is placed over the affected area.

If Lidex is applied to a wide area of the body for prolonged periods, the drug may be absorbed through the skin and cause additional problems.

What should you know about the drug?
If Lidex causes local irritation of the skin, its use should be discontinued.

Skin infections do not respond to Lidex. In such cases, an appropriate antibacterial or antifungal agent should first be used to clear the infection. Applying Lidex may cause the infection to spread.

Are there any special precautions?
Use Lidex only under the close supervision of your physician. Do not apply the drug to areas of the skin that seem infected.

The safe use of Lidex during pregnancy has not been established.

Lomotil®

Generic name
This product contains a combination of diphenoxylate hydrochloride and atropine sulfate.

Class of drug
Antidiarrheal

In what form is the drug available?
Tablets and liquid

Why is the drug prescribed?
It is used in the treatment of diarrhea. The drug acts by slowing down the movements of the intestines.

What are some possible side effects?
The most frequently encountered side effects include dry mouth, flushing, dry skin, urinary retention, an increase in the heart rate (tachycardia), nausea, vomiting, dizziness, loss of appetite (anorexia), drowsiness, itching, and abdominal discomfort.

A few patients taking Lomotil may experience euphoria, numbness of the arms and legs, depression, and skin rashes.

What should you know about the drug?
If taken in excessive amounts over prolonged periods, Lomotil may cause psychological or physical dependence. Do not exceed the recommended dose.

Lomotil should be used only for the short-term treatment of diarrhea. The drug should not be given to children under the age of two years.

Oversedation often occurs when Lomotil is taken at the same time as alcohol, tranquilizers, sedatives, or other depressants of the central nervous system.

Are there any special precautions?
Lomotil should be used with extreme caution in persons with cirrhosis and other advanced diseases of the liver. Lomotil may aggravate certain intestinal disorders. Consult a physician if symptoms persist or increase.

Lomotil should be used with caution (if at all) during pregnancy. The drug appears in breast milk during the lactation period, and may affect the nursing infant.

Lo/Ovral®

Generic name
This product contains a combination of norgestrel and ethinyl estradiol.

Class of drug
Oral contraceptive

In what form is the drug available?
Tablets

Why is the drug prescribed?
It is used for the prevention of pregnancy (contraception).

What are some possible side effects?
The most frequently encountered side effects that may result from the use of oral contraceptives are: nausea, bloating, breakthrough bleeding (spotting), abdominal cramps, tenderness of the breasts, headache, vaginal itching, increased vaginal discharge, infection of the vagina, mental depression, fatigue, increased appetite, and weight gain.

Much less common but potentially more serious side effects can occur. These include: the formation of blood clots in deep veins, high blood pressure, gall bladder disease, and an increase in the blood sugar.

Other serious diseases (e.g., breast cancer) are possibly related to taking oral contraceptives, but a clear cause-and-effect relationship remains to be proved.

What should you know about the drug?
Lo/Ovral contains about sixty per cent of the hormones available in Ovral—thus the name Lo (low).

Lo/Ovral, like many oral contraceptives, contains a combination of two synthetic female hormones. Acting together, they inhibit the release of new eggs from the ovary. Thus, ovulation is prevented and pregnancy is avoided. All modern oral contraceptives are extremely effective.

Lo/Ovral contains less estrogen than many other oral contraceptives. This may be associated with a reduced incidence of side effects, although it is also responsible for an increase in breakthrough bleeding (spotting during the middle of the menstrual cycle). Current evidence suggests that Lo/Ovral may be just as effective as oral contraceptives containing higher doses of hormones.

Are there any special precautions?
Oral contraceptives should not be used in women with blood-clotting disorders, thrombophlebitis, heart dis-

ease, disease of the blood vessels of the brain (cerebral vascular disease), coronary artery disease, or in those with a history of these diseases or of myocardial infarction (heart attack).

Oral contraceptives should not be given to women with known or suspected breast cancer, undiagnosed vaginal bleeding, known or suspected pregnancy, or certain forms of liver disease.

Smoking cigarettes increases the risk of serious side effects while taking oral contraceptives. This risk increases both with age (especially in women over thirty-five) and the number of cigarettes smoked daily.

Macrodantin®

Generic name
Nitrofurantoin macrocrystals

Class of drug
Antibacterial (urinary tract only)

In what form is the drug available?
Capsules

Why is the drug prescribed?
It is used to treat specific bacterial infections of the urinary tract, including those that affect the kidneys and bladder.

What are some possible side effects?
The most frequently encountered side effects are loss of appetite (anorexia), nausea, vomiting, and diarrhea. Some patients also experience abdominal pain, skin rashes, itching, drug-induced fever, joint pains, headache, dizziness, and drowsiness.

A few patients taking Macrodantin have experienced more serious side effects. These include: severe allergic reactions (anaphylactic shock), impairment of the blood-forming tissues, and serious disorders of nerve function (peripheral neuropathy).

What should you know about the drug?
Macrodantin is designed to treat only specific bacterial infections of the urinary tract. It has little or no therapeutic effect on other parts of the body.

The drug should not be used in patients with impaired kidney function. It should be used with extreme caution (if at all) in patients with anemia, diabetes, vitamin B deficiency, and serious chronic diseases. In this group of patients, Macrodantin can cause severe or irreversible nerve damage.

Are there any special precautions?
The safe use of Macrodantin during pregnancy has not been established. The drug should not be administered to women of childbearing age unless necessary.

Marax®

Generic name
This product contains a combination of ephedrine sulfate, theophylline, and hydroxyzine hydrochloride.

Class of drug
Bronchodilator/antiasthmatic

In what form is the drug available?
Tablets and syrup

Why is the drug prescribed?
It is used to prevent or relieve the symptoms of asthma or other breathing disorders associated with spasm or constriction of the lower air passages (bronchial tubes). Marax helps open up (dilate) the lower air passages.

What are some possible side effects?
The most frequently encountered side effects include nervousness, high blood pressure (hypertension), increased heart rate (tachycardia), a sensation of the heartbeat (palpitations), irregular heart rhythms (cardiac arrhythmias), sweating, headache, a feeling of warmth, and dryness of the nose and throat.

Some patients while taking Marax also experience stomach irritation, particularly if the drug is taken on an empty stomach, nausea, vomiting, abdominal discomfort, and retention of urine.

What should you know about the drug?
The FDA, based partly on a review of the drug by the National Academy of Sciences, states that Marax is "possibly" effective for controlling bronchospastic disorders.

Marax should *not* be used in patients with heart disease, increased activity of the thyroid gland (hyperthyroidism), and high blood pressure (hypertension). It should be used with caution in elderly males with known disease of the prostate gland.

Drowsiness can be a problem when Marax is taken with alcohol, sedatives, tranquilizers, or other depressants of the central nervous system. Use caution when driving, operating potentially dangerous machinery, or engaging in other activities that require mental alertness until the effects of the drug are known for a particular individual.

Are there any special precautions?

The manufacturer warns that Marax should *not* be used during early pregnancy. It should be used with extreme caution (if at all) during later stages of pregnancy.

Experimental studies with rats have shown that Marax can cause fetal abnormalities in these animals at doses substantially above the human therapeutic level.

Consult your physician before taking any other drugs at the same time as Marax.

Medrol® Tablets

Generic name
Methylprednisolone

Class of drug
Corticosteroid (synthetic glucocorticoid)

In what form is the drug available?
Tablets

Why is the drug prescribed?
It is used in the treatment of a wide variety of inflammatory and allergic conditions.

Medrol also is used, especially in combination with other corticosteroids, in the treatment of disorders of the adrenal glands to replace hormones normally produced by these glands.

What are some possible side effects?
Corticosteroids, including Medrol, can cause a broad

range of adverse effects. These effects are related to the dose prescribed and the duration of therapy. The age and general condition of the patient can also influence the type and severity of side effects.

Among the possible side effects of Medrol therapy are: water retention resulting in swelling of the tissues (edema); weakness; the accumulation of fatty deposits around the face, neck, or abdomen; weight gain; increased susceptibility to bruising; upset stomach; peptic ulcer; suppressed growth in children; depression; nervousness; euphoria; insomnia; skin changes; a decrease in the density of bones (osteoporosis), leading to an increased risk of fractures; and an increased susceptibility to fungal, bacterial, and viral infections.

What should you know about the drug?
Medrol, like all other corticosteroids, is an extremely potent drug. Its use must be under the close supervision of your physician.

Dosage requirements vary greatly from patient to patient. Even in a particular individual, the amount of Medrol given may have to be modified during the course of therapy. This depends on the disease being treated and the response of the patient.

Report any side effects to your physician at once.

Are there any special precautions?
Medrol Tablets should be used with caution (if at all) during pregnancy and during the nursing period.

Patients taking Medrol should not be vaccinated against smallpox or be subjected to any other immunization procedures.

Consult your physician before taking any other drugs at the same time as Medrol Tablets.

Mellaril®

Generic name
Thioridazine hydrochloride (phenothiazine group)

Class of drug
Major tranquilizer

In what form is the drug available?
Tablets and solution (taken by mouth)

Why is the drug prescribed?

It is used to relieve the symptoms of depression, anxiety, aggression, and agitation associated with severe mental illnesses (psychoses).

The manufacturer also claims that Mellaril is effective in treating the symptoms of alcohol withdrawal and severe (intractable) pain.

What are some possible side effects?

The manufacturer claims that, when Mellaril is given in the recommended dosage, most side effects are mild and temporary.

Side effects reported in patients taking Mellaril include drowsiness, dry mouth, blurred vision, constipation, nausea, vomiting, diarrhea, stuffy nose (nasal congestion), pallor, loss of appetite (anorexia), and menstrual irregularities.

Some patients taking Mellaril or other drugs in this class have experienced skin rashes, swelling of the tissues caused by fluid retention (edema), drug-induced fever, asthma, jaundice, restlessness, muscular rigidity, and symptoms that resemble Parkinsonism (fixed facial expression and shaking or trembling of the limbs). A few patients have experienced confusion, hyperactivity, psychotic reactions, and impairment of the blood-forming tissues.

What should you know about the drug?

The FDA, based partly on a review of this drug by the National Academy of Sciences, states that Mellaril is "effective" in the treatment of psychotic disorders and "probably effective" in the management of moderate to severe aggressiveness, agitation, or hyperactivity in disturbed children.

The FDA considers Mellaril "possibly effective" in the treatment of symptoms associated with alcohol withdrawal and severe (intractable) pain.

Are there any special precautions?

Consult your physician before taking any other drugs at the same time as Mellaril. Oversedation can occur if this drug is taken at the same time as alcohol, sedatives, or other depressants of the central nervous system.

Mellaril should be used with caution (if at all) during pregnancy.

meprobamate

Brand names
Equanil® Miltown®

Class of drug
Minor tranquilizer

In what form is the drug available?
Tablets and capsules

Why is the drug prescribed?
It is used mainly to relieve mild anxiety and tension.
The drug may also help induce sleep in persons who
are anxious and tense at bedtime.

What are some possible side effects?
The most frequently encountered side effects include
drowsiness, impairment of muscular coordination
(ataxia), dizziness, slurred speech, weakness, headache, overstimulation, visual disturbances, nausea,
vomiting, diarrhea, increased heart rate (tachycardia),
a sensation of the heartbeat (palpitations), skin rashes,
and itching.

Some patients taking meprobamate have experienced a severe drop in blood pressure (hypotension),
disturbances in heart rhythms (cardiac arrhythmias),
severe allergic reactions (anaphylactic shock), and
impairment of the blood-forming tissues. Physical and
psychological dependence can develop with prolonged
use.

What should you know about the drug?
Meprobamate is an ingredient of several fixed-
combination drug products. The effects of meprobamate are similar in most ways to those of barbiturates.

Meprobamate was originally developed as a muscle
relaxant, and the drug was once prescribed for its
anticonvulsant properties. It is no longer considered
effective for such purposes. Meprobamate can aggravate a certain form of epilepsy (grand mal seizures).
Sudden withdrawal of the drug, especially in patients
who have been receiving relatively high doses, can
induce convulsions.

Are there any special precautions?
Meprobamate may impair mental alertness, especially

when taken at the same time as alcohol or other depressants of the central nervous system. Extreme caution must be taken when driving or operating potentially dangerous machinery until the drug's effects on a particular individual are established.

Meprobamate should be used with extreme caution (if at all) during pregnancy and lactation (the nursing period). There is a possible risk of fetal malformation with the use of minor tranquilizers, including meprobamate.

Monistat®

Generic name
Miconazole nitrate

Class of drug
Antifungal agent

In what form is the drug available?
Vaginal cream

Why is the drug prescribed?
It is used to treat a specific fungal (yeast) infection of the vagina and external genitals. The infection is known as candidiasis (formerly, moniliasis).

What are some possible side effects?
The most frequently encountered side effects are itching, burning, or irritation of the vagina or external genitals (vulva). A few patients also experience skin rashes, pelvic cramps, and headache.

What should you know about the drug?
The manufacturer claims that Monistat is effective in all women whether or not they are pregnant, or taking oral contraceptives. However, it should be used during the first three months of pregnancy only if it is absolutely necessary to insure the welfare of the patient.

Monistat must be taken exactly as prescribed. Otherwise, there is a danger of recurring infections.

Are there any special precautions?
Discontinue the use of Monistat and consult your physician if irritation or sensitization occurs.

Motrin®

Generic name
Ibuprofen

Class of drug
Anti-inflammatory

In what form is the drug available?
Tablets

Why is the drug prescribed?
It is used to provide symptomatic relief of pain and disability associated with two specific types of joint inflammation (rheumatoid arthritis and osteoarthritis).

What are some possible side effects?
The most frequently encountered side effects include nausea, indigestion (including heartburn), abdominal cramps or pain, diarrhea, constipation, bloating, flatulence, dizziness, headache, and itching.

Some patients taking Motrin also experience a ringing in the ears (tinnitus), a loss of appetite (anorexia), fluid retention with swelling of the tissues (edema), skin rashes, and impairment of vision.

What should you know about the drug?
The manufacturer claims that the effectiveness of Motrin has been demonstrated by the reduction in joint swelling, pain, duration of morning stiffness, and disease activity. Greater functional ability is shown by an increase in grip strength and a delay in the time it takes to tire.

Are there any special precautions?
Motrin should be used with extreme caution in patients with heart failure (cardiac decompensation), a history of peptic ulcer, and in those with blood-clotting abnormalities. Signs of bleeding or visual changes should be reported to your physician at once.

Motrin should not be used during pregnancy or by nursing mothers.

Consult your physician before taking any other drugs at the same time as Motrin.

Mycolog®

Generic name
This product contains a combination of nystatin, neomycin sulfate, gramicidin, and triamcinolone acetonide.

Class of drug
Antibiotic/antifungal/anti-inflammatory

In what form is the drug available?
Cream and ointment

Why is the drug prescribed?
The manufacturer claims that Mycolog is useful in the treatment of specific bacterial and fungal infections of the skin. The FDA, based partly on a review of the drug by the National Academy of Sciences states that the cream form of the drug is "possibly effective" in the relief of itching of the anus and female external genital organs (vulva), when caused by a bacterial or fungal infection.

What are some possible side effects?
The most frequently encountered side effects are itching, burning sensations, irritation, and dry skin. The skin condition being treated may be made worse if the patient is sensitive (experiences an allergic reaction) to any of the ingredients of Mycolog. This is often the case with the neomycin ingredient, which has a relatively high incidence of allergic reactions.

Mycolog should not be used to treat virus infections of the skin such as chicken pox or shingles, since it may spread the infection or make it worse.

Mycolog should not be applied to large areas. The drug may be absorbed through the skin and cause kidney damage or impair hearing.

What should you know about the drug?
The antifungal ingredient of Mycolog is specific for the treatment of a yeastlike infection known as candidiasis (formerly known as moniliasis).

Prolonged use of Mycolog may result in the overgrowth of various species of microorganisms both bacterial and fungal.

Are there any special precautions?

If local skin irritation is noted during the use of Mycolog, discontinue its use and consult your physician immediately.

Mycostatin® Vaginal Tablets

Generic name
Nystatin

Class of drug
Antifungal agent

In what form is the drug available?
Tablets (for insertion into the vagina)

Why is the drug prescribed?
It is used mainly to treat localized fungus infections of the vagina and external genitals of women, especially those fungi *Candida albicans,* which cause the disease known as candidiasis (formerly moniliasis).

What are some possible side effects?
The manufacturer states that Mycostatin is virtually nonpoisonous and nonsensitizing, and is well tolerated by women of all ages, even during long periods of treatment. Minor irritations occasionally occur.

What should you know about the drug?
No adverse effects or complications have been reported in children born to women treated with Mycostatin Vaginal Tablets during their pregnancies.

Are there any special precautions?
If irritation of the genital area is experienced during the use of Mycostatin Vaginal Tablets, discontinue the use of the drug and consult your physician.

Naldecon®

Generic name
This product contains a combination of phenylpropanolamine hydrochloride, phenylephrine hydrochloride, phenyltoloxamine citrate, and chlorpheniramine maleate.

Class of drug
Antihistamine and decongestant

In what form is the drug available?
Syrup, tablets, pediatric drops, and pediatric syrup

Why is the drug prescribed?
It is used to relieve nasal congestion associated with allergies such as hay fever (allergic rhinitis), the common cold, and sinusitis.

What are some possible side effects?
The most frequently encountered side effects are drowsiness, blurred vision, and difficulty urinating.

Some patients taking Naldecon may experience a sensation of the heartbeat (palpitations), an increase in the heart rate (tachycardia), and—if taken for prolonged periods—a chronic runny nose. Nasal congestion may recur if it is suddenly discontinued.

What should you know about the drug?
Naldecon should be used with caution in patients with high blood pressure (hypertension), heart disease, thyroid disease, diabetes, glaucoma, and disease of the prostate gland.

Are there any special precautions?
Avoid using Naldecon if you are pregnant or a nursing mother. Naldecon should not be taken by children under twelve years of age.

Nalfon®

Generic name
Fenoprofen calcium

Class of drug
Anti-inflammatory

In what form is the drug available?
Capsules and tablets

Why is the drug prescribed?
It is used to provide symptomatic relief of pain and disability associated with rheumatoid arthritis and osteoarthritis.

What are some possible side effects?

The most frequently encountered side effects include upset stomach or dyspepsia (in about one out of every seven patients), constipation, nausea, vomiting, abdominal pain, loss of appetite (anorexia), traces of blood in the stools, diarrhea, flatulence, and dry mouth.

Sleepiness and headache occur in approximately one out of every seven patients. Itching and a ringing in the ears occur in approximately one out of every ten patients. About two out of every fifty patients experience a sensation of the heartbeat (palpitations).

Less frequently encountered side effects include a general feeling of being unwell (malaise), skin rashes, increased sweating, dizziness, tremor, mental confusion, nervousness, difficulty urinating, insomnia, blurred vision, and an increase in the heart rate (tachycardia).

What should you know about the drug?

The manufacturer claims that the effectiveness of Nalfon in patients with rheumatoid arthritis is shown by the reduction in joint swelling, pain, duration of morning sickness, and disease activity. Greater mobility of the joints is also achieved. Similar effects are claimed when Nalfon is used in the treatment of osteoarthritis.

Nalfon should be used with caution in patients with a known history of disease of the upper part of the digestive tract.

Are there any special precautions?

Nalfon should not be used during pregnancy or by nursing mothers.

Naprosyn®

Generic name
Naproxen

Class of drug
Anti-inflammatory

In what form is the drug available?
Tablets

Why is the drug prescribed?

It is used to provide symptomatic relief of pain and disability associated with rheumatoid arthritis.

What are some possible side effects?

The most frequently encountered side effects include nausea, upset stomach (including heartburn), abdominal pains, constipation, diarrhea, vomiting, traces of blood in the stools, headache, drowsiness, dizziness, lightheadedness, mental confusion, and depression.

Some patients taking Naprosyn have experienced itching (pruritus), skin rashes, increased sweating, visual disturbances, a ringing in the ears (tinnitus), edema, and a sensation of the heartbeat (palpitations).

On rare occasions, a few patients also have had jaundice and impairment of the blood-forming tissues.

What should you know about the drug?

Severe and occasionally fatal bleeding from the digestive tract has occurred in some patients taking Naprosyn. This drug should be used with extreme caution (if at all) in patients with active peptic ulcers or diseases of the stomach or intestines.

Are there any special precautions?

Naprosyn should not be used during pregnancy or by nursing mothers.

Consult your physician before taking any other drugs at the same time as Naprosyn.

Neosporin®

Generic name

This product contains a combination of polymyxin B sulfate, neomycin sulfate, and gramicidin.

Class of drug

Topical antibiotic (for use in the eye)

In what form is the drug available?

Solution (for application with eyedropper), ointment

Why is the drug prescribed?

It is used for the short-term treatment of bacterial infections of the eye.

What are some possible side effects?

The most frequently encountered side effect is local irritation of the eye after application of Neosporin.

What should you know about the drug?

Neosporin Ophthalmic Solution contains a combination of three antibiotics, which exert broad-spectrum activity. Ideally, of course, eye infections should be treated with an antibiotic that is specific for the microorganism involved.

   If the eye infection shows no signs of improvement after a few days of therapy with Neosporin Ophthalmic Solution or ointment, consult your physician.

Are there any special precautions?

Neosporin Ophthalmic Solution should not be used in any person with a known sensitivity (allergic reaction) to any of its ingredients.

nitroglycerin

Brand names

Cardabid® Nitro-Bid® Nitroglyn® Nitrol® Nitrong® Nitrospan® Nitrostat®

Class of drug

Antianginal agent

In what form is the drug available?

Capsules and tablets, and ointment or paste for application to the skin where it is absorbed over a prolonged period

Why is the drug prescribed?

It is used in the treatment of patients with angina pectoris to decrease the frequency and severity of chest pain. The pain is the result of a temporarily insufficient supply of blood to the heart muscle through the coronary arteries.

What are some possible side effects?

Among the possible side effects experienced by patients taking nitroglycerin, or any of the brand names listed above, are the following: headache, dizziness, flushing, a drop in blood pressure after suddenly standing up from a sitting or reclining position (postural hypotension), sensation of the heartbeat (palpitations), increased heart rate (tachycardia), nausea, vomiting, skin rashes, blurred vision, dry mouth, restlessness, pallor, increased sweating, weakness, and collapse.

What should you know about the drug?

Nitroglycerin is most commonly administered as sublingual tablets (a form which dissolves and is absorbed when placed under the tongue).

If the prescribed dose of nitroglycerin, which can be up to three tablets taken during one attack, does not relieve anginal pain, consult your physician at once.

Nitroglycerin tends to lose its effectiveness if stored for prolonged periods. Some authorities say that the potency of nitroglycerin begins to fade after one to three months, while others suggest that the drug may remain effective for much longer periods. One sign of the drug's freshness is a burning or stinging sensation when placed under the tongue (applicable only to the sublingual tablets).

Are there any special precautions?

If the pain is not relieved within approximately fifteen minutes, consult your physician immediately. There is a danger that the cause may not be angina pectoris but symptoms of an acute myocardial infarction.

Norgesic®

Generic name

This product contains a combination of orphenadrine citrate, aspirin, phenacetin, and caffeine.

Class of drug

Analgesic

In what form is the drug available?

Tablets

Why is the drug prescribed?

It is used mainly to relieve mild to moderate muscular pains.

What are some possible side effects?

The most frequently encountered side effects include

dry mouth, blurred vision, nausea, vomiting, headache, dizziness, constipation, drowsiness, difficulty urinating, an increase in the heart rate (tachycardia), and
a sensation of the heartbeat (palpitations).

Some patients taking Norgesic may experience hives
and other skin eruptions.

What should you know about the drug?

Prolonged or excessive use of the phenacetin ingredient in Norgesic can cause kidney damage.

The aspirin ingredient of Norgesic can cause stomach irritation or bleeding in patients who are especially sensitive to the effects of this common pain reliever.

The orphenadrine ingredient of Norgesic can cause
drowsiness, which can be increased by simultaneously
taking alcohol, tranquilizers, or other depressants of
the central nervous system. Use caution when engaging in any tasks that require mental alertness.

It is claimed that Norgesic exerts its intended therapeutic effects by helping reduce muscular rigidity and
spasm, and by relieving associated pain.

Because of the possibility of adverse effects when the
two drugs are taken at the same time, patients being
treated with Norgesic should not be given Darvon.

Are there any special precautions?

Norgesic should not be given to patients with glaucoma, obstruction of the neck of the bladder, disease of
the prostate gland, or obstruction of the passage from
the exit of the stomach to the small intestine. Safety of
the drug's administration during pregnancy or to children has not yet been established.

Consult your physician before taking any other
drugs at the same time as Norgesic.

Norinyl®

Generic name
This product contains a combination of norethindrone
and mestranol.

Class of drug
Oral contraceptive

In what form is the drug available?
Tablets

Why is the drug prescribed?

It is used for the prevention of pregnancy (contraception).

What are some possible side effects?

The most frequently encountered side effects that may result from the use of oral contraceptives are: nausea, bloating, vaginal bleeding, abdominal cramps, tenderness of the breasts, headache, vaginal itching, increased vaginal discharge, infection of the vagina, depression, fatigue, increased appetite, and weight gain.

Much less common but potentially more serious side effects can occur. These include: formation of blood clots in deep veins, high blood pressure (hypertension), gall bladder disease, and an increase in the blood sugar.

Other serious diseases (e.g., breast cancer) are possibly related to taking oral contraceptives. However, a clear cause-and-effect relationship remains to be proved.

What should you know about the drug?

Norinyl, like many other oral contraceptives, contains a combination of two synthetic female hormones. Acting together, they inhibit the release of eggs from the ovary. Thus, ovulation is prevented and pregnancy is avoided.

Are there any special precautions?

Oral contraceptives should not be used in women with blood-clotting disorders, thrombophlebitis, heart disease, disease of the blood vessels of the brain (cerebral vascular disease), coronary artery disease, or in those with a history of these diseases or of myocardial infarction (heart attack).

Oral contraceptives should not be given to women with known or suspected breast cancer, undiagnosed vaginal bleeding, known or suspected pregnancy, or certain forms of liver disease.

Smoking cigarettes increases the risk of serious side effects while taking oral contraceptives. This risk increases both with age (especially in women over thirty-five) and the number of cigarettes smoked daily.

Norlestrin-21®

Generic name
This product contains a combination of norethindrone acetate and ethinyl estradiol.

Class of drug
Oral contraceptive

In what form is the drug available?
Tablets

Why is the drug prescribed?
It is used for the prevention of pregnancy (contraception).

What are some possible side effects?
The most frequently encountered side effects that may result from the use of oral contraceptives are: nausea, bloating, vaginal bleeding, abdominal cramps, tenderness of the breasts, headache, vaginal itching, increased vaginal discharge, infection of the vagina, depression, fatigue, increased appetite, and weight gain.

Much less common but potentially more serious side effects can occur. These include: the formation of blood clots in deep veins, high blood pressure, gall bladder disease, and an increase in the blood sugar.

Other serious diseases (e.g., breast cancer) are possibly related to taking oral contraceptives, but a clear cause-and-effect relationship remains to be proved.

What should you know about the drug?
Norlestrin-21, like many oral contraceptives, contains a combination of two synthetic female hormones. Acting together, they inhibit the release of new eggs from the ovary. Thus, ovulation is prevented and pregnancy is avoided. All modern oral contraceptives are extremely effective.

Are there any special precautions?
Oral contraceptives should not be used in women with blood-clotting disorders, thrombophlebitis, heart disease, disease of the blood vessels of the brain (cerebral vascular disease), coronary artery disease, hypertension, or in those with a history of these diseases or of myocardial infarction (heart attack).

Oral contraceptives should not be given to women with known or suspected breast cancer, undiagnosed vaginal bleeding, known or suspected pregnancy, or certain forms of liver disease.

Smoking cigarettes increases the risk of serious side effects while taking oral contraceptives. This risk increases both with age (especially in women over thirty-five) and the number of cigarettes smoked daily.

Orinase®

Generic name
Tolbutamide

Class of drug
Oral hypoglycemic (antidiabetic) agent

In what form is the drug available?
Tablets

Why is the drug prescribed?
It is used in the treatment of selected patients with diabetes, usually those with a relatively mild form of the disease. The majority of patients able to benefit from this class of drug (which is *not* insulin) experience the first signs of diabetes toward middle age (maturity-onset diabetes). The drug is of no value if the patient's pancreas is unable to manufacture insulin.

What are some possible side effects?
The most frequently encountered side effect is a severe *drop* in the level of sugar (glucose) in the blood. This condition is known as hypoglycemia. The patient becomes confused, weak, dizzy, and may break out in a cold sweat. In severe cases, when immediate medical attention is required, the patient may lapse into a coma.

Less common side effects include abnormalities of the blood or liver, skin rashes, and retention of water in the tissues which causes swelling (edema).

What should you know about the drug?
A potentially dangerous drop in the level of blood sugar may occur if Orinase is taken together with certain other drugs. These include: antibacterial sul-

fonamides, phenylbutazone, salicylates (e.g., aspirin), probenecid, dicoumarol, and MAO inhibitors.

Thiazide diuretics (water pills) may reduce the effects of Orinase.

Orinase should not be used to treat juvenile or growth-onset diabetes, severe or unstable (brittle) diabetes, or diabetes accompanied by various complications.

The drug should not be given to patients about to undergo major surgery, those with severe infections, or those who have suffered severe injuries.

Are there any special precautions?

If adverse effects are experienced while taking Orinase, consult your physician immediately.

Ornade®

Generic name

This product contains a combination of chlorpheniramine maleate, phenylpropanolamine hydrochloride, and isopropamide iodide.

Class of drug

Antihistamine and decongestant

In what form is the drug available?

Capsules

Why is the drug prescribed?

It is used to relieve nasal congestion (stuffy nose) and runny nose, especially when caused by hay fever (allergic rhinitis). The manufacturer also claims that Ornade is useful in relieving nasal congestion and drying up excess secretions (hypersecretion) when caused by the common cold or sinusitis.

What are some possible side effects?

The most frequently encountered side effects include drowsiness and excessive dryness of the nose, throat, or mouth. Some patients taking Ornade may also experience nervousness or insomnia.

Less frequently encountered side effects include nausea, vomiting, abdominal discomfort or pain, diarrhea, weakness, dizziness, irritability, a sensation of the heartbeat (palpitations), difficulty urinating, a change in blood pressure, constipation, and visual disturbances.

A few patients taking Ornade have experienced convulsions and impairment of the blood-forming tissues.

What should you know about the drug?

The FDA, based partly on a review of this drug by the National Academy of Sciences, states that Ornade is "possibly effective" for the relief of upper respiratory tract congestion and hypersecretion associated with hay fever (allergic rhinitis) and similar conditions in which the cause is not an allergic reaction. The FDA states that Ornade is "lacking in substantial evidence of effectiveness" for relief of symptoms associated with the common cold and sinusitis.

Are there any special precautions?

Ornade must be used with caution in persons with heart disease, glaucoma, disease of the prostate gland, and an overactive thyroid gland (hyperthyroidism).

Ortho-Novum®

Generic name

This product contains a combination of norethindrone and mestranol.

Class of drug

Oral contraceptive

In what form is the drug available?

Tablets

Why is the drug prescribed?

It is used for the prevention of pregnancy (contraception).

What are some possible side effects?

The most frequently encountered side effects that may result from the use of oral contraceptives are: nausea, bloating, vaginal bleeding, abdominal cramps, tenderness of the breasts, headache, vaginal itching, increased vaginal discharge, infection of the vagina, depression, fatigue, increased appetite, and weight gain.

Much less common but potentially more serious side effects can occur. These include: the formation of blood clots in deep veins, high blood pressure, gall bladder disease, and an increase in the blood sugar.

Other serious diseases (e.g., breast cancer) are possibly related to taking oral contraceptives, but a clear cause-and-effect relationship remains to be proved.

What should you know about the drug?

Ortho-Novum, like many oral contraceptives, contains a combination of two synthetic female hormones. Acting together, they inhibit the release of new eggs from the ovary. Thus, ovulation is prevented and pregnancy is avoided. All modern oral contraceptives are extremely effective.

Are there any special precautions?

Oral contraceptives should not be used in women with blood-clotting disorders, thrombophlebitis, heart disease, disease of the blood vessels of the brain (cerebral vascular disease), coronary artery disease, or in those with a history of these diseases or of myocardial infarction (heart attack).

Oral contraceptives should not be given to women with known or suspected breast cancer, undiagnosed vaginal bleeding, known or suspected pregnancy, or certain forms of liver disease.

Smoking cigarettes increases the risk of serious side effects while taking oral contraceptives. This risk increases both with age (especially in women over thirty-five) and the number of cigarettes smoked daily.

Ovral®

Generic name

This product contains a combination of norgestrel and ethinyl estradiol.

Class of drug

Oral contraceptive

In what form is the drug available?

Tablets

Why is the drug prescribed?

It is used to prevent pregnancy (contraception).

What are some possible side effects?

The most frequently encountered side effects are: increased appetite, weight gain, nausea, bloating, breakthrough bleeding (spotting), abdominal cramps, tenderness of the breasts, headache, vaginal itching, increased vaginal discharge, infection of the vagina, mental depression, and fatigue.

Much less common but potentially more serious side effects can occur. These include: the formation of blood clots in deep veins, high blood pressure, gall bladder disease, and an increase in the blood sugar.

Other serious diseases (e.g., breast cancer) are possibly related to taking oral contraceptives, but a clear cause-and-effect relationship remains to be proved.

What should you know about the drug?

Ovral contains more of the hormones available in the companion product Lo/Ovral.

Ovral, like many oral contraceptives, contains a combination of two synthetic female hormones. Acting together, they inhibit the release of new eggs from the ovary. Thus, ovulation is prevented and pregnancy is avoided. All modern oral contraceptives are extremely effective.

Are there any special precautions?

Oral contraceptives should not be used in women with blood-clotting disorders, thrombophlebitis, heart disease, disease of the blood vessels of the brain (cerebral vascular disease), coronary artery disease, or in those with a history of these diseases or of myocardial infarction (heart attack).

Oral contraceptives should not be given to women with known or suspected breast cancer, undiagnosed vaginal bleeding, known or suspected pregnancy, or certain forms of liver disease.

Smoking cigarettes increases the risk of serious side effects while taking oral contraceptives. This risk increases both with age (especially in women over thirty-five) and the number of cigarettes smoked daily.

Ovulen®

Generic name

This product contains a combination of ethynodiol diacetate and mestranol.

Class of drug
Oral contraceptive

In what form is the drug available?
Tablets

Why is the drug prescribed?
It is used to prevent pregnancy (contraception).

What are some possible side effects?
The most frequently encountered side effects that may result from the use of oral contraceptives are: nausea, bloating, vaginal bleeding, abdominal cramps, increased vaginal discharge, infection of the vagina, depression, fatigue, increased appetite, and weight gain.

Much less common but potentially more serious side effects can occur. These include: the formation of blood clots in deep veins, high blood pressure, gall bladder disease, and an increase in the blood sugar.

Other serious diseases (e.g., breast cancer) are possibly related to taking oral contraceptives, but a clear cause-and-effect relationship remains to be proved.

What should you know about the drug?
Ovulen, like many oral contraceptives, contains a combination of two synthetic female hormones. Acting together, they inhibit the release of new eggs from the ovary. Thus, ovulation is prevented and pregnancy is avoided. All modern oral contraceptives are extremely effective.

Are there any special precautions?
Ovulen should not be used in women with blood-clotting disorders, thrombophlebitis, heart disease, disease of the blood vessels of the brain (cerebral vascular disease), coronary artery disease, or in those with a history of these diseases or of myocardial infarction (heart attack).

Oral contraceptives should not be given to women with known or suspected breast cancer, undiagnosed vaginal bleeding, known or suspected pregnancy, or certain forms of liver disease.

Smoking cigarettes increases the risk of serious side effects while taking oral contraceptives. This risk increases both with age (especially in women over thirty-five) and the number of cigarettes smoked daily.

114

Parafon Forte®

Generic name
This product contains a combination of chlorzoxazone and acetaminophen.

Class of drug
Skeletal muscle relaxant and analgesic

In what form is the drug available?
Tablets

Why is the drug prescribed?
It is used to relieve the discomfort of painful muscle spasm, particularly of the back or neck.

What are some possible side effects?
The manufacturer claims that after more than two decades of extensive clinical use of products that contain chlorzoxazone, that drug has been shown to be well tolerated and rarely produces any adverse effects. However, some patients taking Parafon Forte, this combination drug product, may become drowsy or dizzy, or may experience disturbances and, in rare cases, bleeding of the digestive tract.

Other reported side effects include lightheadedness, overstimulation, and a general feeling of being unwell (malaise). A few patients taking this drug may note a reddish-purple discoloration of the urine. This finding is of no known medical significance.

What should you know about the drug?
The FDA, based partly on a review of this drug by the National Academy of Sciences, states that Parafon Forte is "probably effective" as a contributing means of relief, when combined with rest and physical therapy, of discomfort associated with "acute, painful musculo-skeletal conditions."

Chlorzoxazone, the skeletal muscle relaxant in Parafon Forte, does not directly relax tense skeletal muscles in humans. Some experts believe that the effectiveness of Parafon Forte is largely the result of its painkilling acetaminophen ingredient.

Prolonged use of Parafon Forte, especially in large doses, increases the possible risk of liver damage.

Are there any special precautions?

This drug should be used with caution (if at all) during pregnancy, or in women who are likely to become pregnant.

Discontinue the use of Parafon Forte at the first sign of an allergic reaction, such as hives or itching of the skin. Consult your physician at once if this occurs.

Pavabid®

Generic name

Papaverine hydrochloride

Class of drug

Vasodilator

In what form is the drug available?

Capsules

Why is the drug prescribed?

This drug is designed to increase the flow of blood in the arms, legs, heart, and brain by relaxing the muscular walls of the blood vessels (vasodilator action). It is used in conditions where spasm of the arteries impairs the blood flow to these areas.

What are some possible side effects?

Possible adverse reactions in patients taking Pavabid include nausea, abdominal discomfort, loss of appetite (anorexia), constipation, a general feeling of being unwell (malaise), drowsiness, dizziness, increased sweating, headache, diarrhea, skin rashes, flushing of the face, an increase in the heart rate and the depth of respiration, and a slight increase in blood pressure (hypertension). A few patients taking Pavabid may also experience jaundice and impairment of liver function.

What should you know about the drug?

The American Medical Association in its publication *AMA Drug Evaluations,* states that Pavabid is of questionable effectiveness as an oral drug, and that "the place of this agent in therapy has not been clearly established."

Are there any special precautions?

Pavabid should be used with caution (if at all) in persons with glaucoma.

There is little if any justification to use this drug during pregnancy or during the nursing period, especially since its effectiveness is uncertain.

penicillin G

Brand names

Bicillin® Pentids® Pfizerpen G® Sk-Penicillin G® Sugracillin® Wycillin®

Class of drug

Antibiotic

In what form is the drug available?

Tablets, oral solution, and injectable

Why is the drug prescribed?

It is used to treat a wide variety of bacterial infections.

What are some possible side effects?

Allergic reactions are the most frequently encountered side effects in patients taking any of the various forms of penicillin. In those who are particularly sensitive (hypersensitive) to this class of drug, penicillin can cause a severe and potentially fatal reaction (anaphylactic shock). Although allergic reactions can occur with any dosage form, they are more common when the drug is injected. Less severe allergic reactions include skin rashes, joint pains, and fever.

Penicillin can also cause a disturbance of the normal bacterial population of the digestive tract. This promotes an overgrowth of one or more species of microorganisms. An example of the result of such a superinfection is inflammation of the lining of the mouth (stomatitis) and the tongue (glossitis). When taken orally, the most frequently encountered side effects are an upset stomach, cramps, and diarrhea.

What should you know about the drug?

Penicillin was first discovered in 1928. But it was not until the 1940s that it was widely used to treat bacterial infections. Penicillin G was the original form of penicillin introduced into medical practice. Many physicians still consider it as the drug of choice to control infections caused by a large number of bacteria. Penicillins are not effective against fungi or viruses.

Slightly different chemical forms of penicillin G are available. All have about the same ability to interfere with the metabolism of the cell walls of susceptible bacteria and thus prevent the spread of infection.

The effectiveness of the oral forms of penicillin G can be impaired by natural stomach acids. The absorption of the drug into the body can also be impaired if food is in the stomach.

When taking any antibiotic it is essential to follow the physician's instructions to the letter. Don't stop taking the drug just because you feel better. Complete the full course of therapy. Failure to do this may result in a flare-up of the infection a few days later. It also may result in bacterial resistance to the drug which would make its later use ineffective against the same bacteria.

Are there any special precautions?

Penicillin G should never be given to anyone with a known allergic reaction to it or to other forms of penicillin. There is also a greater chance that an adverse reaction will occur if the patient has a general history of other allergies such as hay fever, asthma, or hives.

penicillin VK

Brand names

Betapen VK® Ledercillin VK® Pen-Vee K® Pfizerpen VK® Robicillin VK® SK-Penicillin VK® Uticillin VK® V-Cillin K® Veetids®

Class of drug

Antibiotic

In what form is the drug available?

Tablets and oral solution

Why is the drug prescribed?

It is used to treat a wide variety of bacterial infections.

What are some possible side effects?

Allergic reactions are the most frequently encountered side effects in patients taking any form of penicillin. In those who are particularly sensitive (hypersensitive) to this class of drug, penicillin can cause a severe and potentially fatal reaction (anaphylactic shock). Other possible allergic reactions to penicillin include skin rashes, joint pains, and fever.

When taken orally, the most frequently encountered side effects of penicillin are an upset stomach, cramps, and diarrhea.

What should you know about the drug?

Penicillin VK is available only in oral forms. Its major advantage over penicillin G (see above) is that it is more resistant to the effects of natural stomach acids. Thus, it is more readily absorbed into the body. The antibacterial effectiveness of penicillin VK is similar to that of penicillin G.

When taking any antibiotic it is essential to follow the physician's instructions to the letter. Don't stop taking the drug just because you feel better. Complete the full course of therapy. Failure to do this may result in a flare-up of the infection a few days later. It also may result in bacterial resistance to the drug which would make its later use ineffective against the same bacteria.

Are there any special precautions?

Penicillin VK should never be given to anyone with a known allergic reaction to it or to other forms of penicillin. There is also a greater chance that an adverse reaction will occur if the patient has a general history of other allergies such as hay fever, asthma, or hives.

Percodan®

Generic name

This product contains a combination of oxycodone hydrochloride, oxycodone terephthalate, aspirin, phenacetin, and caffeine.

Class of drug

Narcotic analgesic

In what form is the drug available?
Tablets

Why is the drug prescribed?
It is used for the relief of moderate to moderately
severe pain.

What are some possible side effects?
The most frequently encountered side effects include
lightheadedness, dizziness, nausea, vomiting, and sedation. In some patients these reactions may be relieved by lying down.

Some patients taking Percodan may also experience
euphoria, constipation, and itching (pruritus).

What should you know about the drug?
The oxycodone hydrochloride and oxycodone terephthalate ingredients of Percodan are narcotic analgesics
(painkillers). Thus, the drug can be habit-forming,
especially if taken for prolonged periods. In cases of
overdose, these ingredients can cause a decrease in
breathing rate (respiratory depression), coma, stopping
of the heart (cardiac arrest), shock, and death.

Other possible side effects in patients taking Percodan include nausea, constipation, stomach irritation
or bleeding, kidney damage, and occasional allergic
reactions.

The sedative effects of Percodan can be increased by
taking alcohol, tranquilizers, or other depressants of
the central nervous system. Use caution when driving,
operating potentially dangerous machinery, or engaging in other tasks that demand mental alertness until
the effects of the drug are known for an individual
patient.

Are there any special precautions?
Percodan should be used with extreme caution (if at
all) during pregnancy. Its possible effects on the developing fetus are not known.

The full-strength form of Percodan should not be
given to children. Percodan®-Demi is available, and
contains half the amount of narcotic analgesics as
Percodan.

Percodan should be used with caution (if at all) in
patients with stomach ulcers, impaired kidney function, and blood-clotting abnormalities.

Periactin®

Generic name
Cyproheptadine hydrochloride

Class of drug
Antihistamine (plus antiserotonin action)

In what form is the drug available?
Tablets and syrup

Why is the drug prescribed?
It is used mainly to relieve the symptoms of hay fever (allergic rhinitis), allergic conjunctivitis, allergic inflammations of the skin (allergic dermatitis), and to improve the condition in patients who have experienced an allergic reaction to a transfusion of blood or plasma.

What are some possible side effects?
The most frequently encountered side effects include sleepiness, sedation, dryness of the mouth, nose and throat, thickening of the secretions in the lower air passages (bronchial tubes), abdominal discomfort, and impairment of muscular coordination.

Some patients taking this class of drug may experience nervousness, confusion, fatigue, nausea, vomiting, diarrhea, constipation, wheezing, skin rashes, blurred vision, a ringing in the ears (tinnitus), headache, a sensation of the heartbeat (palpitations), an increase in the heartbeat (tachycardia), stuffy nose, difficulty urinating, excessive perspiration, loss of appetite (anorexia), and a drop in blood pressure (hypotension).

A few patients may experience potentially more serious side effects. These include: convulsions, severe allergic reactions (anaphylactic shock), and impairment of the blood-forming tissues.

What should you know about the drug?
Overdosage with Periactin, particularly in infants and children, can cause hallucinations, convulsions, and death.

The sedative effects of Periactin can be increased by taking alcohol, tranquilizers, or other substances that depress the central nervous system. Use caution when driving, operating potentially dangerous machinery, or engaging in other tasks that demand mental alertness until the drug effects on a patient are known.

Are there any special precautions?
Periactin should be used with extreme caution (if at all) during pregnancy. The drug should *not* be used by nursing mothers.

Periactin should be used with caution in patients with a history of bronchial asthma, glaucoma, heart disease, increased activity of the thyroid gland (hyperthyroidism), and high blood pressure (hypertension).

Persantine®

Generic name
Dipyridamole

Class of drug
Antianginal agent/coronary vasodilator

In what form is the drug available?
Tablets

Why is the drug prescribed?
It is used in the long-term treatment of patients with angina pectoris to decrease the frequency and severity of chest pain. The pain is the result of a temporarily insufficient supply of blood through the coronary arteries to the heart muscle.

What are some possible side effects?
The manufacturer claims that when Persantine is taken at recommended dosages, the adverse effects experienced are mild and of no real duration. The most frequently encountered of these side effects are headache, dizziness, nausea, flushing, weakness, upset stomach, and skin rash.

What should you know about the drug?
Persantine, unlike nitroglycerin, is not designed to provide immediate relief of pain during an attack of angina pectoris.

The FDA, based partly on a review of the drug by the National Academy of Sciences, states that Persantine is "possibly effective" for long-term therapy of chronic angina pectoris.

The manufacturer claims that no particular contra-indications have been reported in the use of Persantine.

Are there any special precautions?

Persantine should be used with caution in patients who have an abnormally low blood pressure (hypotension). Excessive doses of the drug can cause an additional lowering of blood pressure, which could prove dangerous.

Phenaphen® with Codeine

Generic name

This product contains a combination of codeine phosphate and acetaminophen.

Class of drug

Narcotic analgesic

In what form is the drug available?

Capsules

Why is the drug prescribed?

It is used for the relief of mild to moderate pain.

What are some possible side effects?

The most frequently encountered side effects include lightheadedness, dizziness, sedation, nausea, and vomiting. These effects can often be relieved if the patient lies down.

Some patients taking Phenaphen with Codeine may also experience euphoria, constipation, and itching (pruritus).

What should you know about the drug?

The codeine phosphate ingredient of this product may be habit-forming, especially if taken for prolonged periods.

The sedative effects of Phenaphen with Codeine may be increased by taking alcohol, tranquilizers, or other substances that depress the central nervous system. Use caution when driving, operating potentially dangerous machinery, or engaging in other tasks that demand mental alertness until the effects of the drug on an individual patient are known.

Are there any special precautions?

Codeine or any drug containing codeine can be addictive. Overdosage can lead to serious complications. Take Phenaphen with Codeine exactly as prescribed. Report any adverse effects immediately.

Phenergan® Expectorant (Plain)

Generic name

This product contains a combination of promethazine hydrochloride, potassium guaiacolsulfonate, sodium citrate, citric acid anhydrous, ipecac fluid extract, and alcohol.

Class of drug

Antihistamine and expectorant

In what form is the drug available?

Liquid (to be taken by mouth)

Why is the drug prescribed?

It is used to relieve the symptoms of the common cold and some allergies that affect the upper respiratory tract.

What are some possible side effects?

The antihistamine ingredient in Phenergan Expectorant can cause drowsiness in some patients. The expectorant ingredients can cause nausea. (Expectorants act to loosen the secretions in the lower air passages and promote their expulsion naturally or by means of the cough reflex.)

What should you know about the drug?

The sedative effects of Phenergan Expectorant can be increased by taking alcohol, tranquilizers, or other substances that depress the central nervous system. Use caution when driving, operating potentially dangerous machinery, or engaging in other tasks that require mental alertness until the effects on an individual patient are known.

Are there any special precautions?

Phenergan Expectorant should be used with caution (if at all) during pregnancy and during the nursing period.

Phenergan® Expectorant with Codeine

Generic name

This product contains a combination of codeine phosphate, promethazine hydrochloride, potassium guaiacolsulfonate, sodium citrate, citric acid anhydrous, ipecac fluid extract, and alcohol.

Class of drug

Cough suppressant (antitussive), antihistamine, and expectorant

In what form is the drug available?

Liquid (to be taken by mouth)

Why is the drug prescribed?

It is used to suppress coughing and to relieve the symptoms of the common cold and some allergies that affect the upper respiratory tract.

What are some possible side effects?

The most frequently encountered side effects include drowsiness, dry mouth, difficulty urinating, blurred vision, nausea, and constipation. Some patients may also experience a sensation of the heartbeat (palpitations) and nervousness.

What should you know about the drug?

The codeine phosphate in this product may be habit-forming, especially if taken for prolonged periods.

The sedative effects of Phenergan Expectorant with Codeine can be increased by taking alcohol, tranquilizers, or other substances that depress the central nervous system. Use caution when driving, operating potentially dangerous machinery, or engaging in other tasks that require mental alertness until the effects of the drug are known in an individual patient.

Are there any special precautions?

Codeine or any drug containing codeine can be addictive. Overdosage can lead to serious complications. Take Phenergan Expectorant with Codeine exectly as prescribed by your physician. Report any adverse effects immediately.

Consult your physician before taking any other drugs at the same time as this product.

Phenergan Expectorant with Codeine should be used with caution (if at all) during pregnancy and during the nursing period.

Phenergan® VC Expectorant (Plain)

Generic name
This product contains a combination of phenylephrine hydrochloride, promethazine hydrochloride, potassium guaiacolsulfonate, sodium citrate, citric acid, ipecac fluid extract, and alcohol.

Class of drug
Decongestant, antihistamine, and expectorant

In what form is the drug available?
Liquid (to be taken by mouth)

Why is the drug prescribed?
It is used to relieve stuffy nose (nasal congestion) and other symptoms associated with the common cold and some allergies that affect the upper respiratory tract.

What are some possible side effects?
The most frequently encountered side effects include drowsiness, dryness of the nose, mouth, and throat, nausea, nervousness, a sensation of the heartbeat (palpitations), blurred vision, and constipation.

What should you know about the drug?
This product contains the same ingredients as Phenergan Expectorant (Plain), with the addition of the decongestant ingredient phenylephrine hydrochloride. (See above.)

The sedative effects of Phenergan VC Expectorant can be increased by taking alcohol, tranquilizers, or other substances that act to depress the central nervous system. Use caution when driving, operating potentially dangerous machinery, or engaging in other tasks that require mental alertness until the effects of the drug on an individual patient are known.

Are there any special precautions?
Phenergan VC Expectorant should be used with caution (if at all) during pregnancy and during the nursing period.

Phenergan® VC Expectorant with Codeine

Generic name

This product contains a combination of codeine phosphate, phenylephrine hydrochloride, promethazine hydrochloride, potassium guaiacolsulfonate, sodium citrate, citric acid, ipecac fluid extract, and alcohol.

Class of drug

Cough suppressant (antitussive), decongestant, antihistamine, and expectorant

In what form is the drug available?

Liquid (to be taken by mouth)

Why is the drug prescribed?

It is used to suppress coughing and to relieve stuffy nose (nasal congestion) and other symptoms associated with the common cold and some allergies that affect the upper respiratory tract.

What are some possible side effects?

The most frequently encountered side effects include drowsiness, dryness of the nose, mouth, and throat, difficulty urinating, blurred vision, nausea, a sensation of the heartbeat (palpitations), nervousness, and constipation.

What should you know about the drug?

This product contains the same ingredients as Phenergan VC Expectorant (Plain), with the addition of the narcotic ingredient codeine phosphate. (See above.)

The sedative effects of Phenergan VC Expectorant with Codeine can be increased by taking alcohol, tranquilizers, or other substances that depress the central nervous system. Use caution when driving, operating potentially dangerous machinery, or engaging in other tasks that demand mental alertness until the effects of the drug on an individual patient are known.

The codeine phosphate ingredient in this product can be habit-forming, especially if taken for prolonged periods.

Are there any special precautions?

Codeine or any drug containing codeine can be addictive. Overdosage can lead to serious complications. Take Phenergan VC Expectorant with Codeine exactly as prescribed by your physician. Report any adverse effects immediately. Consult your physician before taking any other drugs with this product.

Phenergan VC Expectorant with Codeine should be used with caution (if at all) during pregnancy and during the nursing period.

phenobarbital

Brand names

Luminal® SK-Phenobarbital® Solfoton®

Class of drug

Sedative, hypnotic (sleeping pill), and anticonvulsant

In what form is the drug available?

Tablets, capsules, and elixir (to be taken by mouth)

Why is the drug prescribed?

It is used, alone or in combination with other drugs, to relieve mild tension and chronic anxiety (sedative action), induce sleep (hypnotic action), and control convulsive seizures (anticonvulsant action).

What are some possible side effects?

The most frequently encountered side effects include: drowsiness; depression; dizziness; difficulty in breathing; nausea; vomiting; diarrhea; hangover, especially in the morning when phenobarbital has been used the night before to induce sleep in patients with insomnia; and allergic reactions such as skin rashes.

What should you know about the drug?

Phenobarbital is a member of the general class of drugs known as barbiturates. Prolonged use of these drugs can lead to physical dependence.

Overdosage with phenobarbital can be extremely serious. It is a major cause of drug-induced deaths, especially in persons with suicidal tendencies. The sedative effects of phenobarbital can be greatly increased by taking alcohol, tranquilizers, or other substances that depress the central nervous system.

Consult your physician before taking any other drugs at the same time as phenobarbital, or any combination product that contains phenobarbital.

Are there any special precautions?

Do not take any alcoholic drinks during the period of therapy with phenobarbital. The combined effects can be hazardous and potentially fatal.

Safe use of phenobarbital during pregnancy and the nursing period has not been established.

Phenobarbital should be used with caution (if at all) in patients with a history of liver or kidney disease.

Persons with porphyria or a history of porphyria (a rare disorder caused by an inborn error of metabolism) must *not* take phenobarbital or other barbiturates. Such drugs can bring on an attack.

Poly-Vi-Flor®

Generic name

This product contains a combination of vitamins A, B_6, B_{12}, C, D, E, folic acid, thiamine, riboflavin, niacin, plus fluoride.

Class of drug

Multivitamin supplement with a fluoride

In what form is the drug available?

Liquid (dispensed with a dropper) and chewable tablets

Why is the drug prescribed?

It is used in children to correct vitamin deficiencies and to prevent or minimize dental cavities.

What are some possible side effects?

The manufacturer states that allergic rash and any other unusual reactions have rarely been reported with the use of Poly-Vi-Flor. However, when certain vitamins—such as vitamins A and D—are taken in excessive amounts, they tend to accumulate in the body. Such a build-up of vitamins can cause toxic (poisonous) effects.

Other side effects that may occur with the use of Poly-Vi-Flor include stomach upset, headache, weakness, and itching (pruritus).

What should you know about the drug?

Supplementary vitamins are usually not needed if you eat well-balanced meals, with generous amounts of fresh fruit and vegetables.

The fluoride ingredient of Poly-Vi-Flor is designed to prevent the formation of dental cavities. However, in areas with a natural availability of fluoride in the drinking water—or in areas where fluoride is added to the drinking water of the community—Poly-Vi-Flor should not generally be used. An excessive amount of fluoride can be harmful.

Are there any special precautions?

The manufacturer warns that Poly-Vi-Flor should not be used if the drinking water contains fluoride (in excess of 0.7 parts per million).

Do not exceed the dosage recommended by your physician. Prolonged use of large amounts of fluoride can damage the teeth.

prednisone

Brand names

Deltasone® Meticorten® Orasone® Sterapred®

Class of drug

Corticosteroid (synthetic glucocorticoid)

In what form is the drug available?

Tablets

Why is the drug prescribed?

It is used in the treatment of a wide variety of inflammatory and allergic conditions.

In combination with other corticosteroids, prednisone is also used in the treatment of disorders of the adrenal glands, such as Addison's disease, to replace the hormones normally produced by these glands.

What are some possible side effects?

Corticosteroids, including prednisone, can cause a broad range of adverse effects. These are especially related to the dose prescribed and the duration of therapy. The age and general condition of the patient can also influence the type and severity of side effects.

The following are examples of the side effects associated with prednisone therapy: water retention, resulting in swelling of the tissues (edema); weakness, resulting from the loss of the mineral potassium; the accumulation of deposits of fat around the face (moon face), neck (buffalo hump), or abdomen; increased susceptibility to bruising; weight gain; stomach upset; peptic ulcer; suppressed growth in children; reactivation of tuberculosis; personality changes, including euphoria and depression; nervousness; irritability; insomnia; various changes in the appearance of the skin; a decrease in the density of bones (osteoporosis), leading to an increased risk of fractures; and an increased susceptibility to various fungal, bacterial, and viral infections.

What should you know about the drug?

Prednisone, like all other corticosteroids, is an extremely potent drug. Its use must be under the close supervision of your physician.

Dosage requirements vary greatly from person to person. Even in a particular patient, the amount of prednisone given may have to be modified during the course of therapy depending on the disease being treated and the patient's response to the drug.

During the period of prednisone therapy, report any side effects to your physician at once.

Are there any special precautions?

Patients taking prednisone should not be vaccinated against smallpox or be subjected to any other immunization procedures.

Consult your physician before taking any other drugs at the same time as prednisone.

Prednisone should be used with caution (if at all) during pregnancy and the nursing period.

Premarin®

Generic name
Conjugated estrogen

Class of drug
Mixture of estrogen female hormone compounds

In what form is the drug available?

Tablets (a vaginal cream and an injectable form are also available)

Why is the drug prescribed?

One of its main uses is to relieve some of the symptoms associated with menopause (change of life). However, the manufacturer cautions that estrogens should not be used in the treatment of nervous symptoms or depression as there is no proof of their effectiveness in conditions such as these.

Premarin is also used to replace estrogen deficiencies in women following surgical removal of the ovaries, the natural source of female hormones.

Other conditions in which Premarin may provide relief include: various types of menstrual disorders, failure of the ovaries to secrete hormones, breast swelling following childbirth, and, in selected cases, as part of the overall treatment of breast cancer, and cancer of the prostate gland in men.

What are some possible side effects?

The most frequently encountered side effects include abdominal discomfort, nausea, weight changes, swelling of the tissues as the result of water retention (edema), changes in mood, headache, vaginal bleeding (spotting), and enlargement of the breasts.

Taking any estrogens, including Premarin, may increase the risk of cancer of the lining of the uterus (endometrial carcinoma), especially in women who have passed menopause. An increased risk of other types of cancer has also been associated with the prolonged use of estrogens, although a clear cause-and-effect relationship remains to be proved.

What should you know about the drug?

The manufacturer warns that Premarin has been shown to be ineffective for the treatment of any condition present during pregnancy and that its use may have a serious effect on the developing fetus.

The use of Premarin may increase the risk of gall bladder disease and the formation of blood clots in deep veins. In general, the possible adverse effects associated with the use of Premarin are similar to those associated with the prolonged use of oral contraceptives.

Are there any special precautions?

Premarin should *not* be used (1) during pregnancy or in women who may be pregnant; (2) in women who have undiagnosed vaginal bleeding; (3) in women with known or suspected breast cancer (except in highly selected cases); (4) in women with blood-clotting abnormalities or a history of such disorders.

Pro-Banthine®

Generic name
Propantheline bromide

Class of drug
Anticholinergic (antispasmodic) agent

In what form is the drug available?
Tablets

Why is the drug prescribed?
It is used mainly in the treatment of the irritable bowel syndrome (irritable colon, spastic colon, mucous colitis), and acute enterocolitis (inflammation of the moist lining of the intestinal tract).

Pro-Banthine is also used as part of the overall therapy for patients with peptic ulcers.

What are some possible side effects?
The most frequently encountered side effects include dry mouth, decreased sweating, blurred vision, an increase in pressure within the eyeball (intraocular tension), urinary retention, an increase in the heart rate (tachycardia), a sensation of the heartbeat (palpitations), loss of the sense of taste, headache, nervousness, mental confusion, drowsiness, weakness, dizziness, insomnia, nausea, vomiting, constipation, and a bloated feeling.

Some patients taking Pro-Banthine may also have an inability to achieve and maintain an erection of the penis (impotence), skin rashes, and may experience a severe allergic reaction to the drug (anaphylactic shock).

What should you know about the drug?
Pro-Banthine works by reducing spasm and normal muscular movements of the stomach and intestines

(antispasmodic action). It also helps to reduce the acid secretions of the stomach, which can be beneficial in treating patients with peptic ulcers.

The use of antacids at the same time as Pro-Banthine can increase the risk of constipation.

Are there any special precautions?

If Pro-Banthine is taken when the environmental temperature is unusually high, there is a possible risk of heatstroke. This can occur because one of the side effects of the drug is to reduce the normal sweating response. This limits the body's ability to regulate the temperature of the skin surface.

Pro-Banthine should be used with caution in the elderly and in persons with disease of the kidneys or liver. It should also be used cautiously in those who have an overactive thyroid gland (hyperthyroidism), heart disease, or high blood pressure (hypertension).

The safe use of Pro-Banthine during pregnancy and the nursing period has not yet been established.

Proloid®

Generic name
Thyroglobulin

Class of drug
Purified thyroid extract (obtained from hogs)

In what form is the drug available?
Tablets

Why is the drug prescribed?
It is used as hormonal replacement therapy in persons with an underactive thyroid gland (hypothyroidism).

What are some possible side effects?
The most frequently encountered side effects are those associated with overdosage. Taking excessive amounts of Proloid can cause side effects that are similar to the signs and symptoms of an overactive thyroid gland (hyperthyroidism). These include: nervousness, menstrual irregularities, sweating, irregular and rapid heartbeat, and angina pectoris (chest pains caused by a temporarily inadequate supply of blood to the heart muscle).

What should you know about the drug?

Massive overdosage with Proloid can lead to extremely serious side effects, including those that are a direct threat to life. Take this drug exactly as prescribed by your physician and report any adverse effects at once.

Proloid should not be used as a means of weight control. This is a misuse of a potent drug.

Are there any special precautions?

Proloid should be used with extreme caution (if at all) in patients with heart disease or angina pectoris.

Consult your physician before taking any other drugs at the same time as Proloid.

Pronestyl®

Generic name
Procainamide hydrochloride

Class of drug
Antiarrhythmic agent

In what form is the drug available?
Capsules and tablets (an injectable form is also available)

Why is the drug prescribed?
It is used to control abnormal and irregular heart rhythms (arrhythmias).

What are some possible side effects?
Large doses of Pronestyl may cause nausea, loss of appetite (anorexia), skin rashes, and itching (pruritus). Some patients may experience mental depression, giddiness, diarrhea, bitter taste, weakness, and severe emotional disturbances (psychosis) with hallucinations.

Potentially more serious side effects have been reported in a few patients taking Pronestyl. These include: signs and symptoms resembling a disease known as lupus erythematosus (chills, fever, joint pains, and facial rash), and severe impairment of the blood-forming tissues.

What should you know about the drug?
People who are known to be allergic to the dental

anesthetic Novocain (procaine) may also be allergic to
Pronestyl.

Consult your physician before taking any other
drugs at the same time as Pronestyl, especially those
which can have a stimulating effect on the heart.
These include various nonprescription products used to
treat coughs, colds, or allergies.

Are there any special precautions?

Advise your physician immediately if you experience
any signs or symptoms of side effects while taking
Pronestyl such as a sore mouth, throat, or gums, or
unexplained fever.

Provera®

Generic name

Medroxyprogesterone acetate

Class of drug

Progestin (female sex hormone)

In what form is the drug available?

Tablets

Why is the drug prescribed?

It is used mainly to treat women who experience
irregular menstrual bleeding not caused by disease or
some known physical disorder such as fibroids, and
painful menstruation.

What are some possible side effects?

Women taking this class of drug may experience
breakthrough bleeding (spotting), swelling of the tissues caused by water retention (edema), changes in
weight, jaundice, skin rashes, itching, and mental
depression.

Among other possible side effects are the formation
of blood clots in deep veins, excessive hair growth on
the body (hirsutism), changes in sex drive (libido), loss
of scalp hair, headache, fatigue, and backache.

What should you know about the drug?

Provera is a synthetic derivative of progesterone, a
female hormone produced by the ovaries and by the
placenta during pregnancy.

Are there any special precautions?

The manufacturer warns that Provera should not be used during the first four months of pregnancy. It should be used with caution (if at all) during later periods of pregnancy.

Provera should *not* be used in women with undiagnosed vaginal bleeding, blood-clotting disorders, liver disease, known or suspected breast cancer, cancer of the genitals, or in those with a history of stroke (cerebral apoplexy).

Detectable amounts of Provera have been noted in the breast milk of nursing mothers. The effect of this on a nursing infant has not yet been determined.

Pyridium®

Generic name
Phenazopyridine hydrochloride

Class of drug
Analgesic (urinary tract)

In what form is the drug available?
Tablets

Why is the drug prescribed?
It is used to relieve the symptoms of pain and burning caused by infection or irritation of the lower part of the urinary tract (bladder and urethra).

What are some possible side effects?
Pyridium may occasionally cause stomach upsets or other disturbances of the digestive tract. Potentially more serious side effects are uncommon unless the patient takes an overdose of the drug. This can result in a form of anemia and damage to the kidneys and liver.

What should you know about the drug?
Pyridium may discolor the urine reddish-orange. This is harmless and has absolutely no medical significance. Once the drug has been discontinued, the urine will return to its normal color.

If the skin or whites of the eyes turn yellow while taking Pyridium, it may be a sign that the kidneys are not working properly. In such cases the drug may accumulate in the body, instead of being flushed out in the urine. Consult your physician if this occurs.

Are there any special precautions?

Pyridium should not be taken by persons with disease of the kidneys.

Quibron®

Generic name

This product contains a combination of theophylline and glyceryl guaiacolate.

Class of drug

Bronchodilator and expectorant

In what form is the drug available?

Capsules and liquid (to be taken by mouth)

Why is the drug prescribed?

It is used to relieve breathing difficulties associated with bronchial asthma, chronic bronchitis, and pulmonary emphysema (a disease of the lungs).

Quibron exerts its therapeutic effects by relaxing or dilating the smooth muscles that control the diameter of the lower air passages (bronchial tubes).

What are some possible side effects?

The most frequently encountered side effects are those associated with overdosage. They include: nausea, vomiting, abdominal pain, diarrhea, headache, irritability, restlessness, muscle twitching, an increase in the heart rate (tachycardia), a sensation of the heartbeat (palpitations), flushing, a drop in blood pressure (hypotension), and excitability. Reducing dosage can in most cases control these effects, or their severity.

What should you know about the drug?

The manufacturer warns that at the recommended dosage, Quibron should not be taken more often than every 6 hours.

Are there any special precautions?

Consult your physician before taking any other drugs at the same time as Quibron. This includes any drugs available without a prescription, some of which may

add to the effects of Quibron and increase the likeli-
hood of an adverse reaction.

quinidine sulfate

Brand names
Quinidex Extentabs® Quinora® SK-Quinidine Sulfate®

Class of drug
Antiarrhythmic agent

In what form is the drug available?
Tablets and capsules

Why is the drug prescribed?
It is used to control abnormal and irregular heart
rhythms (arrhythmias).

What are some possible side effects?
The most frequently encountered side effects include
diarrhea, nausea, vomiting, headache, dizziness, a
sensation of the heartbeat (palpitations), ringing in
the ears (tinnitus), and visual disturbances.
   The possibility of side effects increases if quinidine
sulfate is taken in excessive amounts. This can result
in the accumulation of the drug in the body.

What should you know about the drug?
Quinidine sulfate is obtained from the bark of the
cinchona tree. In its purified form it is an extremely
potent drug and should be used only under close
medical supervision.

Are there any special precautions?
Quinidine sulfate should be used with caution in
patients with congestive heart failure, kidney disease,
and in those with digitalis intoxication.
   Consult your physician before taking any other
drugs at the same time as quinidine sulfate.

Regroton®

Generic name
This product contains a combination of chlorthalidone
and reserpine.

Class of drug
Diuretic and antihypertensive

In what form is the drug available?
Tablets

Why is the drug prescribed?
It is used to eliminate the accumulation of excessive amounts of water and salt from the tissues (diuretic action) and to reduce high blood pressure (antihypertensive action). The combined action of the two ingredients in lowering blood pressure in hypertensive patients is greater than if they were taken separately.

What are some possible side effects?
The most frequently encountered side effects include loss of appetite (anorexia), stomach irritation, nausea, vomiting, diarrhea, constipation, stuffy nose (nasal congestion), muscle cramps, dizziness, weakness, headache, drowsiness, and mental depression.

Some patients taking Regroton may experience skin rashes, acute attacks of gout, blurred vision, difficulty urinating, and a drop in blood pressure (hypotension). In rare cases, Regroton may cause impairment of the blood-forming tissues.

What should you know about the drug?
Physicians have been warned that Regroton, a fixed combination drug, is not recommended as initial therapy for patients with hypertension.

The use of Regroton may cause an excessive loss of the essential mineral potassium through the kidneys. This is especially possible if the drug is taken at higher doses or used for prolonged periods. The side effects that occur with diminished levels of potassium in the body can be minimized or avoided by eating foods rich in potassium such as fruit juice, dried fruit, and bananas. The prescribing physician may also administer potassium supplements.

Are there any special precautions?
Regroton should be used with caution in patients with disease of the kidneys or liver.

This drug should be used with caution (if at all) during pregnancy.

Consult your physician before taking any other drugs at the same time as Regroton.

Ritalin®

Generic name
Methylphenidate hydrochloride

Class of drug
Stimulant (central nervous system)

In what form is the drug available?
Tablets

Why is the drug prescribed?
It is used mainly as part of the overall treatment in children who have been diagnosed as having minimal brain dysfunction (MBD). This condition is characterized by a history of a short attention span, impulsiveness, emotional instability, moderate to severe hyperactivity, and a tendency to be easily distracted. The ability to learn may or may not be impaired.

Ritalin is also used to treat people who have narcolepsy, a condition characterized by sudden and recurring attacks of severe drowsiness or sleep.

What are some possible side effects?
The most frequently encountered side effects are nervousness, difficulty sleeping, and decreased appetite. Some patients taking Ritalin may also experience headache, stomach upsets, dizziness, an increase in blood pressure (hypertension), and a sensation of the heartbeat (palpitations). Prolonged or excessive use of Ritalin may result in psychological dependence.

What should you know about the drug?
The manufacturer cautions that Ritalin should not be administered to children under six years of age since its safe use in this age group has not yet been determined.

Ritalin exerts a stimulant effect similar to amphetamines, a group of chemically related drugs once widely prescribed to suppress appetite in persons who are overweight. This was a misuse of an extremely potent drug. Ritalin has a similar potential for drug abuse.

Are there any special precautions?
Ritalin should not be used in the treatment of patients with severe mental depression, or to relieve the symptoms of normal physical fatigue.

This drug should be used with caution in patients with a history of convulsive seizures. Evidence exists that Ritalin may lower the threshold of the onset of seizures in this group.

Ritalin should be used with caution in patients with high blood pressure (hypertension).

The safe use of Ritalin during pregnancy has not yet been determined.

Salutensin®

Generic name

This product contains a combination of hydroflumethiazide and reserpine.

Class of drug

Diuretic and antihypertensive

In what form is the drug available?

Tablets

Why is the drug prescribed?

It is used in the treatment of patients with high blood pressure (hypertension). The hydroflumethiazide ingredient acts to flush out the excessive accumulation of water and salt in the tissues through the kidneys (diuretic action). The reserpine ingredient is thought to exert an effect on nerve endings. This causes the blood vessels to relax, permitting a decrease in resistance to blood flow (antihypertensive action).

What are some possible side effects?

The most frequently encountered side effects include nausea, vomiting, loss of appetite (anorexia), stomach irritation, diarrhea, constipation, muscle cramps, stuffy nose (nasal congestion), dizziness, weakness, headache, drowsiness, and mental depression.

Some patients taking Salutensin may also experience nervousness, mental depression, skin rashes, blurred vision, acute attacks of gout, a decrease in sex drive, itching (pruritus), and a drop in blood pressure. In a few patients, Salutensin may cause impairment of the blood-forming tissues.

What should you know about the drug?

Fixed combination drugs, including Salutensin, are

not recommended as initial therapy for hypertension. The use of Salutensin may cause an excessive loss of the essential mineral potassium through the kidneys. This can occur especially if the drug is taken at higher doses than prescribed or used for prolonged periods. The side effects that typically take place with diminished levels of potassium can be minimized or avoided by eating foods rich in potassium such as fruit juice, dried fruit, and bananas. The prescribing physician may also administer potassium supplements.

Are there any special precautions?

Salutensin should be used with caution in patients with disease of the kidneys or liver. This drug should be used with caution (if at all) in pregnancy.

Consult your physician before taking any other drugs at the same time as Salutensin.

Ser-Ap-Es®

Generic name

This product contains a combination of reserpine, hydralazine hydrochloride, and hydrochlorothiazide.

Class of drug

Diuretic and antihypertensive

In what form is the drug available?

Tablets

Why is the drug prescribed?

It is used in the treatment of patients with high blood pressure (hypertension). The combined effects of the three ingredients in Ser-Ap-Es act to lower elevated blood pressure.

What are some possible side effects?

The most frequently encountered side effects include loss of appetite (anorexia), stomach irritation, nausea, vomiting, cramps, diarrhea, constipation, dizziness, headache, increased sensitivity of the eyes to light (photosensitivity), drug-induced rashes, weakness, restlessness, and blurred vision.

Some patients taking Ser-Ap-Es may experience stuffy nose (nasal congestion), a drop in blood pressure (hypotension), and mental depression.

What should you know about the drug?

Many experts believe that fixed combination drugs, such as Ser-Ap-Es, are far from ideal. When two or more drugs are combined in a fixed dose it prevents the dosage adjustment of a single ingredient.

The manufacturer warns that Ser-Ap-Es is not recommended as initial therapy for patients with hypertension.

The use of Ser-Ap-Es may cause an excessive loss of the essential mineral potassium through the kidneys. This is most likely to occur if the drug is taken at higher doses or used for prolonged periods. The side effects that occur with diminished levels of potassium in the body can be minimized or avoided by eating foods rich in potassium such as fruit juice, dried fruit, and bananas. The prescribing physician may also administer potassium supplements.

Are there any special precautions?

Ser-Ap-Es should be used with caution (if at all) during pregnancy. The drug should not be used by nursing mothers.

Ser-Ap-Es should be used with caution in patients with disease of the kidneys or liver.

Consult your physician before taking any other drugs at the same time as Ser-Ap-Es.

Serax®

Generic name
Oxazepam

Class of drug
Minor tranquilizer

In what form is the drug available?
Capsules and tablets

Why is the drug prescribed?
It is used for the relief of symptoms of emotional tension, anxiety, agitation, and irritability.

Serax is also used to alleviate the symptoms of alcohol withdrawal.

What are some possible side effects?
The most frequently encountered side effects include

drowsiness, dizziness, vertigo, and headache. Some patients taking Serax may experience minor skin rashes, nausea, lethargy, swelling of the tissues (edema) caused by water retention, slurred speech, tremor, and a change in the sex drive (libido).

What should you know about the drug?

As with all tranquilizers, prolonged use—especially in higher than prescribed doses—can result in psychological or physical dependence on the drug.

Are there any special precautions?

Serax may impair mental alertness, especially if taken at the same time as alcohol or other depressants of the central nervous system. Use caution when driving or operating potentially dangerous machinery until the effects of the drug on a particular individual are known.

Serax should be used with extreme caution (if at all) during pregnancy and the nursing period. There is a possible risk of fetal malformation with the use of minor tranquilizers.

Sinequan®

Generic name
Doxepin hydrochloride

Class of drug
Antidepressant

In what form is the drug available?
Capsules and oral concentrate

Why is the drug prescribed?
It is used mainly to relieve symptoms of depression and anxiety. Sinequan also tends to improve sleep patterns in persons with sleep disturbances.

What are some possible side effects?
The most frequently encountered side effects include drowsiness, dizziness, dry mouth, blurred vision, confusion, difficulty urinating, and constipation.

Some patients taking this class of drug occasionally experience high blood pressure (hypertension), a drop in blood pressure (hypotension), disturbances in the heart rhythm (cardiac arrhythmias), drug-induced rashes, and impairment of the blood-forming tissues.

What should you know about the drug?

Sinequan falls within a general group of drugs known as tricyclic antidepressants. These drugs are not considered to be true tranquilizers and should not be prescribed on a casual basis. It usually takes from two to three weeks before their therapeutic effects are experienced.

Are there any special precautions?

Sinequan should not be used in patients with glaucoma or in those who have difficulty urinating.

This drug should not be used in children under twelve years of age, since safe conditions for its use in this group have not been established.

Sinequan must not be taken at the same time as drugs known as monoamine oxidase (MAO) inhibitors or with certain antihypertensive drugs. Otherwise, extremely serious reactions may occur, including high fever, convulsions, and death.

Alcohol, sedatives, tranquilizers, and other depressants of the central nervous system can cause oversedation if taken at the same time as Sinequan. Use caution when driving, operating potentially dangerous machinery, or engaging in other tasks that demand mental alertness until the effects of the drug on a particular individual are known.

Sinequan should be used with caution (if at all) during pregnancy. Its possible effect on the developing fetus has not yet been established.

Slow-K®

Generic name
Potassium chloride

Class of drug
Potassium supplement

In what form is the drug available?
Tablets (sugar-coated in a wax matrix)

Why is the drug prescribed?
The mineral potassium is essential for the normal

functioning of most bodily organs and tissues. For example, it is essential in the transmission of nerve impulses, the contraction of muscles including the heart muscle and skeletal muscles, and the maintenance of normal kidney function.

When the amount of potassium in the body falls below a certain level (potassium depletion), various side effects can occur. These include weakness, fatigue, and a disturbance in the rhythm of the heartbeat. Severe cases of potassium depletion can lead to paralysis and impaired ability of the kidneys to concentrate urine.

Slow-K is designed to prevent potassium depletion in patients taking diuretics (drugs which act to flush out excessive amounts of water and salt through the kidneys). It is also used to replace potassium lost as a consequence of various metabolic and other disorders.

What are some possible side effects?

The most frequently encountered side effects are caused by irritation of the lining of the stomach and intestines. They include nausea, vomiting, abdominal discomfort, and diarrhea. The risk of these adverse effects can often be prevented or minimized by taking Slow-K with meals, instead of on an empty stomach.

The most serious side effects reported in patients taking Slow-K are bleeding from the stomach and intestines and the formation of peptic ulcers. There is also the possibility that taking Slow-K in large doses over prolonged periods can lead to the accumulation of excessive amounts of potassium in the body. This condition is known as hyperkalemia. In advanced cases it can cause potentially fatal complications (cardiac arrest).

What should you know about the drug?

Slow-K must *not* be taken by patients who do not have a depletion of potassium, or by patients who have an excessive amount of potassium in the body (hyperkalemia).

Slow-K is designed to release its active ingredient potassium chloride slowly into the stomach and small intestine. Theoretically, this should avoid severe irritation of the lining of the digestive tract. However, some experts question whether or not this controlled release feature actually works.

Are there any special precautions?

Slow-K must be used with extreme caution in patients with kidney disease, heart disease, or diabetes.

Slow-K should not be used at the same time as diuretic drugs (water pills) that tend to spare the excretion of potassium through the kidneys.

Stelazine®

Generic name
Trifluoperazine hydrochloride

Class of drug
Major tranquilizer/antipsychotic agent (phenothiazine group)

In what form is the drug available?
Tablets (multiple-dose vials and a liquid concentrate are also available for institutional use)

Why is the drug prescribed?
It is used mainly to relieve the symptoms of severe emotional (psychotic) disorders.

Stelazine is also claimed to be useful in controlling excessive anxiety, tension, and agitation in patients with various neurotic disorders.

What are some possible side effects?
The most frequently encountered side effects include drowsiness, dizziness, skin rashes, dry mouth, insomnia, disturbances in the menstrual cycle, fatigue, muscular weakness, loss of appetite (anorexia), and blurred vision.

Some patients taking Stelazine have experienced jaundice and impairment of the blood-forming tissues.

This class of drug can also cause various neuromuscular reactions. These include spasms of the neck muscles, rigidity of the back muscles, difficulty in swallowing, tremors, and convulsions.

Occasionally, patients taking drugs in the class of phenothiazine derivatives, which includes Stelazine, have experienced a severe and sometimes fatal drop in blood pressure and cardiac arrest (a sudden loss of heart function, resulting in cessation of the blood circulation).

What should you know about the drug?

The effects of Stelazine are increased by taking alcohol, sedatives, or other substances that depress the central nervous system. Use caution when driving, operating potentially dangerous machinery, or engaging in other activities that demand mental alertness until the effects of the drug on a particular individual are known.

Are there any special precautions?

The safe use of Stelazine during pregnancy has not been established. Therefore, this drug should be used only if the therapeutic benefits clearly outweigh the possible risk of injury to the developing fetus.

Synalar®

Generic name
Fluocinolone acetonide

Class of drug
Synthetic corticosteroid (anti-inflammatory)

In what form is the drug available?
Cream, ointment, and solution (in plastic squeeze bottles)

Why is the drug prescribed?
It is used topically (on the skin surface) to treat various inflammatory skin disorders.

What are some possible side effects?

The most frequently encountered side effects with the use of topical corticosteroids including Synalar are itching, dry skin, a burning sensation, and skin eruptions. These occur at the site where the drug is applied, and are more common when a tight dressing is placed over the affected area of skin.

If Synalar is applied to a wide area of the body for prolonged periods, the drug may be absorbed through the skin and cause additional problems, some of which are potentially serious.

What should you know about the drug?
If Synalar causes local irritation of the skin, its use should be discontinued.

Skin infections do not respond to Synalar. In such cases an appropriate antibacterial or antifungal agent should first be used to clear the infection. Applying Synalar may cause the infection to spread.

Are there any special precautions?

Use Synalar only under the close supervision of your physician. Do not apply the drug to areas of the skin that seem infected.

The safe use of Synalar during pregnancy has not been established.

Synalgos-DC®

Generic name

This product contains a combination of dihydrocodeine, promethazine hydrochloride, aspirin, phenacetin, and caffeine.

Class of drug

Narcotic analgesic

In what form is the drug available?

Capsules

Why is the drug prescribed?

It is used to relieve moderate to moderately severe pain, in addition to providing a mild sedative effect.

What are some possible side effects?

The most frequently encountered side effects include lightheadedness, dizziness, drowsiness, sedation, nausea, vomiting, constipation, itching (pruritus), skin reactions, and a drop in blood pressure (hypotension).

Some patients taking this combination drug may experience stomach irritation, bleeding of the stomach lining, kidney damage, insomnia, restlessness, excitement, and an increase in the heart rate (tachycardia).

What should you know about the drug?

Synalgos-DC contains the narcotic drug dihydrocodeine. As with any narcotic, the extended use of dihydrocodeine is accompanied by the risk of addiction.

The sedative effects of Synalgos-DC can be increased by taking alcohol, tranquilizers, or other substances that depress the central nervous system. Use caution when driving, operating potentially dangerous machinery, or engaging in other tasks that require mental alertness until the effects of the drug on a particular individual are known.

Are there any special precautions?

Synalgos-DC should be used with caution (if at all) during pregnancy.

Consult your physician before taking any other drugs at the same time as Synalgos-DC.

Synthroid®

Generic name
Levothyroxine sodium

Class of drug
Synthetic thyroid hormone

In what form is the drug available?
Tablets (an injectable form is also available)

Why is the drug prescribed?
It is used as hormonal replacement therapy in persons with an underactive thyroid gland (hypothyroidism).

What are some possible side effects?
The most frequently encountered side effects are those associated with drug overdosage. Taking excessive amounts of Synthroid can cause side effects that are similar to the signs and symptoms of an overactive thyroid gland (hyperthyroidism). These include: nervousness, menstrual irregularities, sweating, irregular and rapid heartbeat, and chest pains (angina pectoris) caused by a temporarily inadequate supply of blood to the heart muscle.

What should you know about the drug?
Massive overdosage with Synthroid can lead to extremely serious side effects, including those that are a direct threat to life. Take this drug exactly as prescribed and report any adverse effects at once.

Are there any special precautions?
Synthroid should be used with extreme caution (if at all) in patients with heart disease or angina pectoris.

Consult your physician before taking any other drugs at the same time as Synthroid.

Tagamet®

Generic name
Cimetidine

Class of drug
Histamine H_2-receptor antagonist (gastric acid inhibitor)

In what form is the drug available?
Tablets (an injectable form is also available)

Why is the drug prescribed?
It is used in the short-term (up to eight weeks) treatment of patients with duodenal ulcers and related disorders of the stomach. Tagamet acts mainly by inhibiting the secretion of stomach acid.

What are some possible side effects?
The most commonly reported side effects (occurring in approximately one out of every 100 patients treated) are: mild and temporary diarrhea, muscular pain, dizziness, and skin rashes.

What should you know about the drug?
Tagamet represents a new therapeutic class of drug. It was first marketed in the United States in August 1977. By September 1979, Tagamet became one of the most frequently prescribed drugs in America.

There may exist the possibility that the use of Tagamet can increase the incidence of stomach cancer. However, to date there is no direct evidence to support this assertion. The FDA has approved the short-term use of Tagamet.

Are there any special precautions?
Tagamet should be used with caution (if at all) during pregnancy and during the nursing period.

This drug should not be used in children under the age of sixteen, unless the prescribing physician believes that the anticipated benefits are greater than the potential risks.

Do not take any other drugs at the same time as

Tagamet (especially anticoagulants) without the knowledge and advice of your physician.

Talwin®

Generic name
Pentazocine hydrochloride

Class of drug
Analgesic

In what form is the drug available?
Tablets (an injectable form is also available)

Why is the drug prescribed?
It is used for the relief of moderate to severe pain.

What are some possible side effects?
The most frequently encountered side effects include nausea, vomiting, stomach upset, constipation, abdominal discomfort or cramps, diarrhea, loss of appetite (anorexia), dry mouth, dizziness, lightheadedness, sedation, headache, alteration of taste, nervousness, irritability, anxiety, difficulty sleeping, and disturbed dreams.

Some patients taking Talwin also experience blurred vision, hallucinations, sweating, flushing, changes in blood pressure, difficulty breathing, difficulty urinating, increase in the heart rate (tachycardia), tingling sensations in the arms and legs, and impairment of the blood-forming tissues. Drug-induced skin rashes may also occur.

What should you know about the drug?
Talwin was originally developed as a potent analgesic without the risk of addiction of narcotic analgesics such as morphine. Unfortunately, this did not prove to be the case. Prolonged and excessive use of Talwin *can* be addictive.

Painful withdrawal symptoms can occur if the use of Talwin is suddenly discontinued.

Are there any special precautions?
Talwin should be used with extreme caution (if at all) in (1) persons with breathing disorders such as bronchial asthma; (2) persons with diseases of the liver or

153

kidneys; (3) pregnant, potentially pregnant, or nursing
women; (4) epileptics; and (5) persons with a history of
mental illness.

Talwin should not be administered to children under
twelve years of age.

Oversedation may occur if Talwin is taken at the
same time as alcohol, tranquilizers, or other substances that depress the central nervous system. Use
caution when driving, operating potentially dangerous
machinery, or engaging in other tasks that require
mental alertness until the effects of the drug on a
particular individual are known.

Tandearil®

Generic name
Oxyphenbutazone

Class of drug
Anti-inflammatory agent

In what form is the drug available?
Tablets

Why is the drug prescribed?
It is used to provide symptomatic relief of pain and
disability associated with a wide variety of severe joint
inflammations. These include: rheumatoid arthritis,
rheumatoid spondylitis, gout (or gouty arthritis), osteoarthritis, psoriatic arthritis, and painful shoulder
such as bursitis of the shoulder.

Tandearil is also used in the relief of certain forms of
vein inflammation (superficial thrombophlebitis).

What are some possible side effects?
This extremely potent drug can cause a variety of side
effects. Because Tandearil cannot *cure* joint diseases—
it only provides symptomatic relief—the potentially
serious and sometimes fatal side effects do not justify
its routine use.

Tandearil can impair the manufacturing of red and
white blood cells by the bone marrow. This occasionally leads to fatal complications such as aplastic anemia.

Other serious side effects reported with the use of
Tandearil include leukemia, fatal and nonfatal inflammation of the liver (hepatitis), severe allergic reactions

(anaphylactic shock), kidney failure, high blood pressure (hypertension), detached retina, hearing loss, convulsions, hallucinations, and severe mental disorders (psychoses).

What should you know about the drug?

Physicians have been warned that patients receiving Tandearil should be given blood tests throughout therapy at intervals of one or, at most, two weeks. This is in addition to other pertinent tests.

Are there any special precautions?

Tandearil is not a drug for casual use. It can be extremely toxic (poisonous). Patients taking this drug should report any adverse effects at once.

Teldrin®

Generic name
Chlorpheniramine maleate

Class of drug
Antihistamine

In what form is the drug available?
Capsules

Why is the drug prescribed?

It is used to provide temporary relief from the symptoms of hay fever (allergic rhinitis) and other allergies that affect the upper respiratory tract.

What are some possible side effects?

The most frequently encountered side effects include sedation, sleepiness, dizziness, disturbed coordination, abdominal discomfort or pain, and thickening of bronchial secretions. Some persons, especially children, may experience excitability.

Other side effects reported with the use of Teldrin include drug-induced rashes, sensitivity of the eyes to light (photosensitivity), excessive sweating, dryness of the mouth, nose, and throat, headache, an increase in the heart rate (tachycardia), a sensation of the heartbeat (palpitations), nausea, vomiting, diarrhea, constipation, difficulty urinating, blurred vision, and ringing in the ears (tinnitus).

A few patients taking Teldrin have been known to experience hysteria, convulsions, and impairment of the blood-forming tissues.

What should you know about the drug?

Oversedation can occur if Teldrin is taken at the same time as alcohol, tranquilizers, or other depressants of the central nervous system. Use caution when driving, operating potentially dangerous machinery, or engaging in other tasks that require mental alertness until the effects of the drug are known in a particular individual.

Are there any special precautions?

Teldrin should be used with caution in patients with high blood pressure (hypertension), heart disease, asthma, glaucoma, overactive thyroid gland (hyperthyroidism), disease of the prostate gland, and diabetes.

Tenuate®

Generic name
Diethylpropion hydrochloride

Class of drug
Anorectic (appetite suppressant)

In what form is the drug available?
Tablets (also available as Tenuate Dospan® in slow-release tablets)

Why is the drug prescribed?
It is used as an aid in the initial treatment of obese (overweight) persons to suppress appetite.

What are some possible side effects?
The most frequently encountered side effects include nervousness, anxiety, dry mouth, headache, dizziness, diarrhea, constipation, increased heart rate (tachycardia), sensation of the heartbeat (palpitations), and a rise in blood pressure (hypertension).

Some patients taking Tenuate may also experience skin rashes, an inability to achieve or maintain an erection of the penis (impotence), a change in sex drive, and mental changes (psychotic episodes).

What should you know about the drug?

Tenuate, or any other appetite suppressant, should not be taken for prolonged periods. The ability of the drug to suppress appetite tends to lessen with continued use. In addition, psychological dependence on the drug often develops.

Many physicians and experts in nutrition consider the use of appetite-suppressant drugs a basically ineffective way to control weight problems. Dietary changes are essential.

Many overweight people think that they have a glandular problem that makes them gain excess weight. In most cases this is only hopeful thinking. The only way for most people to lose weight is to reduce their food intake.

Are there any special precautions?

Tenuate may impair the ability to drive, operate potentially dangerous machinery, or engage in other tasks where mental alertness is essential.

Tenuate should not be taken by people with heart disorders, irregular heart rhythms, or high blood pressure. Also, the drug is not recommended for administration to pregnant women or to children under the age of twelve years.

Consult your physician before taking any other drugs at the same time as Tenuate.

tetracycline

Brand names

Achromycin-V® Panmycin® Retet® Robitet® Sumycin® Tetrex®

Class of drug

Antibacterial, antiamebic, and antirickettsial

In what form is the drug available?

Tablets, capsules, and syrup (an injectable form and ophthalmic preparations are also available)

Why is the drug prescribed?

It is used to treat a wide variety of microbial infections, including those caused by bacteria, certain protozoa, and rickettsiae (microorganisms intermediate in size between bacteria and viruses).

What are some possible side effects?

The American Medical Association, in its publication *AMA Drug Evaluations,* states that, "All tetracyclines have relatively low toxicity at recommended dosage levels." About ten per cent of patients taking tetracycline experience disturbances of the digestive tract. These include nausea, vomiting, diarrhea, flatulence, heartburn, and loss of appetite (anorexia).

Some patients taking tetracycline experience additional side effects associated with a disturbance of the normal bacterial population of the digestive tract. This promotes an overgrowth of one or more species of microorganisms. An example of the result of such a superinfection is inflammation of the lining of the mouth (stomatitis) and the tongue (glossitis). Some women may also experience itching and inflammation of the vagina and external genitals.

A few patients taking tetracycline may have what is known as a photosensitivity reaction when exposed to strong sunlight. This can result in various types of skin eruptions and rashes, which are usually reversible over a period of days or weeks after use of the drug has been discontinued.

Potentially more serious side effects have been reported with the use of tetracycline. These include damage to the liver and kidneys, impairment of the blood-forming tissues, and severe allergic reactions (anaphylactic shock).

The use of tetracycline by children under the age of eight can cause permanent discoloration of the teeth. It can also cause discoloration of teeth in a fetus if the mother takes tetracycline during the last half of pregnancy when the teeth are developing.

What should you know about the drug?

Antacids containing aluminum, calcium, or magnesium impair the absorption of oral forms of tetracycline into the body. Foods and some dairy products can also impair absorption. Thus, it is important to take tetracycline on an empty stomach: one hour before or two hours after meals.

Are there any special precautions?

Tetracycline should *not* be used in pregnancy or during the nursing period.

Consult your physician before taking any other drugs at the same time as tetracycline.

Thorazine®

Generic name
Chlorpromazine

Class of drug
Major tranquilizer (antipsychotic)

In what form is the drug available?
Tablets, capsules, syrup, and suppositories (an injectable form is also available)

Why is the drug prescribed?
It is used mainly to relieve or control the symptoms of severe depression, anxiety, agitation, and aggressiveness associated with severe mental illnesses (psychotic disorders and manic-depression).

Thorazine is also used to control nausea and vomiting, relieve the symptoms of alcohol withdrawal, control restlessness and apprehension prior to surgery, and relieve intractable hiccups.

What are some possible side effects?
The most frequently encountered side effects include drowsiness, dizziness, mental dullness, blurred vision, dry mouth, constipation, and a drop in blood pressure (hypotension), especially when getting up suddenly from a sitting or reclining position.

Some patients taking Thorazine may experience skin rashes, restlessness, an increased heart rate (tachycardia), convulsions, especially in patients with a history of epilepsy, fever, jaundice, and impairment of the blood-forming tissues.

This class of drug can also cause various neuromuscular reactions. These include spasms of the neck muscles, rigidity of the back muscles, and difficulty in swallowing.

Occasionally, patients taking drugs in the class of phenothiazine derivatives such as Thorazine have experienced a severe, and sometimes fatal, drop in blood pressure and cardiac arrest (a sudden loss of heart function, resulting in cessation of the blood circulation).

What should you know about the drug?
The effects of Thorazine are increased by taking alcohol, sedatives, or other substances that depress the

central nervous system. Use caution when engaging in activities that demand mental alertness, such as driving or operating potentially dangerous machinery.

Are there any special precautions?

The safe use of Thorazine during pregnancy has not been established. It should therefore be used only if the therapeutic benefits clearly outweigh the possible risk of injury to the developing fetus.

thyroid

Brand name
Armour Thyroid®

Class of drug
Desiccated thyroid (a purified extract obtained from the thyroid glands of animals)

In what form is the drug available?
Tablets

Why is the drug prescribed?
It is used as hormone replacement therapy in treating patients with a deficiency of the thyroid gland such as hypothyroidism, myxedema, and simple goiter.

What are some possible side effects?
The most frequently encountered side effects occur as the result of overdosage. Taking excessive amounts of thyroid can cause side effects that are similar to the signs and symptoms of an overactive thyroid gland. These include: nervousness, menstrual irregularities, sweating, irregular and rapid heartbeat, and angina pectoris (chest pains caused by a temporarily inadequate supply of blood to the heart muscle).

What should you know about the drug?
The desiccated thyroid gland of animals is the original substance used to treat patients with an underactive thyroid gland (hypothyroidism). Many physicians prefer to use one of the synthetic preparations of thyroid hormone such as Synthroid. However, as the American Medical Association states in its publication, *AMA Drug Evaluations*, "the use of desiccated thyroid is generally satisfactory for many patients."

Different preparations used to treat thyroid gland deficiencies vary in potency. However, all of these substances produce the same therapeutic effects when prescribed in appropriate doses.

It is extremely important to take this drug exactly as prescribed by your physician. Massive overdosage with thyroid can lead to serious side effects, including those that are a direct threat to life.

No substance used to treat thyroid gland deficiencies should be used to treat patients who are overweight. This is a misuse of an extremely potent hormone.

Are there any special precautions?

This preparation should be used with extreme caution (if at all) in patients with heart disease or angina pectoris.

Consult your physician before taking any other drugs at the same time as thyroid.

Tigan®

Generic name

Trimethobenzamide hydrochloride

Class of drug

Antiemetic agent

In what form is the drug available?

Capsules and suppositories (an injectable form is also available)

Why is the drug prescribed?

It is used to control nausea and vomiting. Tigan is also claimed to be effective in preventing or minimizing the symptoms of motion sickness.

What are some possible side effects?

Some patients taking Tigan may experience dizziness, drowsiness, blurred vision, headache, muscle cramps, mental depression, and a drop in blood pressure (hypotension). A few patients may experience skin rashes, jaundice, and impairment of the blood-forming tissues.

In general, however, the incidence of side effects with the use of Tigan is relatively low.

What should you know about the drug?

The sedative effects of Tigan may be increased by taking alcohol, tranquilizers, or other substances that depress the central nervous system. Use caution when driving, operating potentially dangerous machinery, or engaging in other tasks that demand mental alertness.

Are there any special precautions?

The use of Tigan should be discontinued at the first sign of a skin rash or other evidence of an allergic reaction.

Do not take Tigan, for example, tablets left over from an old prescription, unless directed to do so by your physician. The cause of nausea or vomiting must first be diagnosed. Otherwise, the signs and symptoms of a potentially dangerous condition such as an acute attack of appendicitis may be covered up. Extreme caution is recommended in the administration of the drug to children.

Tofranil®

Generic name
Imipramine hydrochloride

Class of drug
Antidepressant

In what form is the drug available?

Tablets (an injectable form is also available)

Why is the drug prescribed?

It is used mainly to relieve the symptoms of depression.

What are some possible side effects?

The most frequently encountered side effects include drowsiness, dizziness, dry mouth, blurred vision, confusion, difficulty urinating, and constipation.

Some patients taking this class of drug occasionally experience high blood pressure (hypertension), a drop in blood pressure (hypotension), disturbances in the heart rhythm (cardiac arrhythmias), drug-induced rashes, and impairment of the blood-forming tissues.

What should you know about the drug?

Tofranil falls within a general class of drugs known as tricyclic antidepressants. These drugs are not considered to be true tranquilizers and should not be prescribed on a casual basis. It usually takes from two to three weeks before their therapeutic effects are experienced.

Tofranil is not recommended for children.

Are there any special precautions?

Tofranil should not be used in patients with glaucoma or in those who have difficulty urinating (urinary retention).

Tofranil must not be taken at the same time as drugs known as monoamine oxidase (MAO) inhibitors. It should not be used with certain antihypertensive drugs. Otherwise, extremely serious reactions may occur, including high fever, convulsions, and death.

Alcohol, sedatives, tranquilizers, and other depressants of the central nervous system can cause oversedation if taken at the same time as Tofranil. Use caution when driving, operating potentially dangerous machinery, or engaging in other tasks that demand mental alertness.

Tofranil should be used with caution (if at all) during pregnancy. Its possible effect on the developing fetus has not yet been established.

Tolectin®

Generic name
Tolmetin sodium

Class of drug
Anti-inflammatory agent

In what form is the drug available?
Tablets

Why is the drug prescribed?
It is used mainly to provide symptomatic relief of pain and disability associated with rheumatoid arthritis and juvenile rheumatoid arthritis.

What are some possible side effects?
The following are the most frequently encountered

side effects reported in patients taking Tolectin: abdominal pain or discomfort, nausea, vomiting, indigestion, heartburn (pyrosis), constipation, peptic ulcer, headache, dizziness, drowsiness, skin rashes, and nervousness.

What should you know about the drug?
Tolectin should be given with caution (if at all) to patients who are allergic to aspirin and other nonsteroid anti-inflammatory drugs.

Tolectin should be used with extreme caution in patients with a history of disease of the upper part of the digestive tract. This drug can cause peptic ulcers and severe bleeding.

Are there any special precautions?
Tolectin should not be given to pregnant women or used during the nursing period.

Tolinase®

Generic name
Tolazamide

Class of drug
Oral hypoglycemic (antidiabetic) agent

In what form is the drug available?
Tablets

Why is the drug prescribed?
It is used in the treatment of selected patients with diabetes; usually those with a relatively mild form of the disease. The majority of patients able to benefit from this class of drug (which is *not* insulin) experience the first signs of diabetes toward middle age (maturity-onset diabetes). The drug is of no value if the patient's pancreas cannot manufacture insulin.

What are some possible side effects?
The most frequently encountered side effect is a severe *drop* in the level of sugar (glucose) in the blood. This condition is known as hypoglycemia. The patient becomes confused, weak, dizzy, and may break out in a cold sweat. For severe cases requiring immediate medical attention, coma may result.

Less common side effects include abnormalities of the blood or liver, skin rashes, and retention of water in the tissues which causes swelling (edema).

What should you know about the drug?

A potentially dangerous drop in the level of blood sugar may occur if Tolinase is taken together with certain other drugs. These include: antibacterial sulfonamides, phenylbutazone, salicylates (e.g., aspirin), probenecid, dicoumarol, and MAO inhibitors.

Thiazide diuretics (water pills) may reduce the effectiveness of Tolinase.

Tolinase should not be used to treat juvenile or growth-onset diabetes, severe or unstable (brittle) diabetes, or diabetes accompanied by various complications.

The drug should not be given to patients about to undergo major surgery, those with severe infections, or those who have suffered severe injuries.

Are there any special precautions?

If adverse effects are experienced while taking Tolinase, consult your physician immediately.

Tranxene®

Generic name
Clorazepate dipotassium

Class of drug
Minor tranquilizer

In what form is the drug available?
Capsules (a tablet form is also available, as Tranxene-SD® and Tranxene-SD Half Strength®)

Why is the drug prescribed?
It is used mainly to relieve anxiety and nervous tension.

What are some possible side effects?
The most frequently encountered side effect is drowsiness. Less frequent side effects include dizziness, various disturbances and upsets of the stomach and intestines, nervousness, blurred vision, dry mouth, headache, and mental confusion.

165

Some patients taking Tranxene may experience insomnia, temporary skin rashes, fatigue, lack of coordination when walking, irritability, double vision (diplopia), depression, and slurred speech.

What should you know about the drug?

Prolonged use of Tranxene, especially in large doses, may cause psychological and physical dependence.

The sedative effects of Tranxene can be increased by taking alcohol, antihistamines, or other substances that depress the central nervous system. Use caution when driving, operating potentially dangerous machinery, or engaging in other tasks that require mental alertness until the effects of the drug on a particular individual are known.

Are there any special precautions?

Tranxene should *not* be used during pregnancy or nursing. Evidence exists that use of drugs in this class carries the risk of malformations of the developing fetus. The drug is not recommended for administration to anyone under the age of eighteen years.

Triavil®

Generic name

This product contains a combination of amitriptyline hydrochloride and perphenazine.

Class of drug

Major tranquilizer and antidepressant

In what form is the drug available?

Tablets

Why is the drug prescribed?

It is used for the relief of symptoms of moderate to severe anxiety, agitation, and depression.

What are some possible side effects?

The side effects that may occur are those that can be caused individually by each of the two ingredients in this combination product. The manufacturer claims that Triavil has not yet demonstrated any adverse effects peculiar to the combination. See Elavil for possible side effects of amitriptyline hydrochloride.

The perphenazine ingredient of Triavil can cause the following additional side effects in some patients: itching, jaundice, severe skin rashes, trembling in the hands, arms, and feet, stiff gait, and a rigid facial expression that resembles the signs and symptoms of Parkinson's disease or Parkinsonism.

What should you know about the drug?

Many experts dislike the use of fixed-combination drugs, such as Triavil. The problem is that dosage adjustment of the separate ingredients to the needs of an individual patient is impossible.

Are there any special precautions?

Triavil must not be taken at the same time as drugs known as monoamine oxidase (MAO) inhibitors. Otherwise, extremely serious reactions may occur, including high fever, convulsions, and death.

Triavil should be used with extreme caution in patients with glaucoma, retention of urine, a history of convulsive seizures, and patients recovering from a recent heart attack.

If Triavil is taken at the same time as alcohol, sedatives, and other depressants of the central nervous system, oversedation can occur. Use caution when driving, operating potentially dangerous machinery, or engaging in other tasks that demand mental alertness.

Triavil should be used with caution during pregnancy. Its possible effect on the developing fetus has not yet been established. The drug is not recommended for administration to children.

Tuss-Ornade®

Generic name

This product contains a combination of caramiphen edisylate, chlorpheniramine maleate, phenylpropanolamine hydrochloride, and isopropamide iodide.

Class of drug

Cough suppressant (antitussive), antihistamine, and decongestant

In what form is the drug available?

Capsules and liquid

Why is the drug prescribed?

It is used to suppress coughs, relieve nasal congestion, and dry up the secretions of a runny nose when caused by hay fever (allergic rhinitis) or similar allergic reactions.

What are some possible side effects?

The most frequently encountered side effects include drowsiness and excessive dryness of the nose, throat, and mouth. Some patients taking Tuss-Ornade may also experience nervousness or insomnia.

Other reported side effects include nausea, vomiting, abdominal pain or discomfort, diarrhea, weakness, dizziness, irritability, a sensation of the heartbeat (palpitations), difficulty urinating, a change in blood pressure, constipation, and visual disturbances.

A few patients taking the ingredients in Tuss-Ornade have experienced convulsions and impairment of the blood-forming tissues.

What should you know about the drug?

This product contains the same ingredients as Ornade, with the addition of the cough suppressant caramiphen edisylate.

The FDA, based partly on a review of this drug by the National Academy of Sciences, states that Tuss-Ornade is "lacking in substantial evidence of effectiveness as a fixed combination" for the claimed therapeutic benefits.

Are there any special precautions?

Tuss-Ornade must be used with caution in persons with heart disease, glaucoma, disease of the prostate gland, and an overactive thyroid (hyperthyroidism).

Tylenol® with Codeine

Generic name

This product contains a combination of codeine phosphate and acetaminophen.

Class of drug

Narcotic analgesic

In what form is the drug available?

Tablets and elixir (a liquid form to be taken by mouth)

Why is the drug prescribed?
It is used for the relief of mild to moderate pain.

What are some possible side effects?
The most frequently encountered side effects include lightheadedness, dizziness, sedation, nausea, and vomiting. These effects can often be relieved if the patient lies down.

Some patients taking Tylenol with Codeine may also experience euphoria, constipation, and itching.

What should you know about the drug?
The codeine phosphate ingredient of this product may be habit-forming, especially if taken for prolonged periods.

The sedative effects of Tylenol with Codeine may be increased by taking alcohol, tranquilizers, or other substances that depress the central nervous system. Use caution when driving, operating potentially dangerous machinery, or engaging in other tasks that demand mental alertness until the effects of the drug on an individual patient are known.

Are there any special precautions?
Codeine or any drug containing codeine can be addictive. Overdosage can lead to serious complications. Take Tylenol with Codeine exactly as prescribed by your physician. Report any adverse effects at once.

Valisone®

Generic name
Betamethasone valerate

Class of drug
Topical synthetic corticosteroid

In what form is the drug available?
Cream, lotion, ointment, and spray (aerosol)

Why is the drug prescribed?
It is applied to the skin surface to treat various types of inflammatory skin conditions.

What are some possible side effects?
The most frequently encountered side effects with the

use of any topical corticosteroids, including Valisone, are itching, dry skin, a burning sensation, and skin eruptions. These occur at the site where the drug is applied, and are more common when a tight dressing is placed over the affected area of skin.

If Valisone is applied to a wide area of the body for prolonged periods, the drug may be absorbed through the skin and cause additional problems, some of which are potentially serious.

What should you know about the drug?

If Valisone causes a local irritation of the skin, discontinue its use.

Skin infections do not respond to Valiscone. In such cases an appropriate antibacterial or antifungal agent should first be used to clear the infection. Applying Valisone may cause the infection to spread.

Are there any special precautions?

Use Valisone only under the close supervision of your physician. Do not apply the drug to areas of the skin that seem infected.

The safe use of Valisone during pregnancy has not been established.

Valium®

Generic name

Diazepam

Class of drug

Minor tranquilizer (with claimed action also as a skeletal muscle relaxant and an anticonvulsant)

In what form is the drug available?

Tablets and as a liquid compounded for injection

Why is the drug prescribed?

The main use of this drug is to relieve symptoms of emotional tension, anxiety, apprehension, and psychoneurotic states brought on by fatigue, agitation, or less severe forms of depression. In the majority of cases the tablet form of the drug is prescribed.

Valium is also prescribed to alleviate symptoms in alcoholics following the sudden withdrawal of alcohol. Such symptoms include shaking (tremors), delirium tremens (d.t.'s), and hallucinations. In addition, Valium has been claimed to be of use in controlling muscular spasms and convulsions when prescribed with certain other drugs.

What are some possible side effects?

The most frequently encountered side effects are drowsiness, a feeling of tiredness or fatigue, and a loss of muscular coordination that can result in unsteadiness when walking. Less often the drug may cause skin rashes of various types, slurred speech, blurred vision, dizziness or fainting, nausea, and an irregularity in menstrual periods.

Reports exist of more serious side effects in patients taking Valium. These include: jaundice; a reduction in the number of circulating white blood cells which leads to an increased susceptibility to bacterial infection; and paradoxical reactions (those which the drug is ordinarily expected to suppress) such as acute excitability, rage, and disordered sleep. In some patients with epilepsy who receive the drug, it tends to increase the frequency and severity of convulsive seizures.

Valium has occasionally been implicated—particularly when injected into a vein—as a causal factor in potentially dangerous falls in blood pressure (hypotension) and in depression of the breathing rate.

What should you know about the drug?

Valium should not be prescribed for patients with a known hypersensitivity (allergic reaction) to it, or for children under the age of six months. Because of the possibility that it may have an adverse effect in patients with a particular form of glaucoma (narrow-angle glaucoma), it should not be prescribed for this group.

The effectiveness of the long-term (more than four months) use of Valium has not been clearly established. The manufacturer suggests that its usefulness for each patient be reassessed periodically.

Are there any special precautions?

The drug should not be taken by pregnant women because its possible effect on the developing fetus has not been established.

Until the effects of the drug on an individual patient are known (the dosage may have to be modified by the prescribing physician), avoid any activity that demands mental alertness such as driving a car or operating potentially dangerous machinery.

Alcoholic drinks may increase the sedative effects of Valium, and the drug may also increase the intoxicating effects of alcohol.

Do not take any other drugs with Valium without the knowledge and advice of your physician.

Vasodilan®

Generic name
Isoxsuprine hydrochloride

Class of drug
Vasodilator

In what form is the drug available?
Tablets (an injectable form is also available)

Why is the drug prescribed?
It is designed to relieve symptoms associated with an inadequate supply of blood to the brain (cerebral vascular insufficiency). Vasodilan is also prescribed to relieve symptoms of an inadequate blood supply to the extremities, including the hands and feet (peripheral vascular disease).

Vasodilan is presumed by the manufacturer to achieve its effects by relaxing blood vessels, thus permitting an increased flow of blood.

What are some possible side effects?
Some patients taking Vasodilan may experience a drop in blood pressure (hypotension), an increase in the heart rate (tachycardia), nausea, vomiting, dizziness, abdominal pain or discomfort, and severe skin rashes.

What should you know about the drug?
The FDA, based partly on a review of the drug by the National Academy of Sciences, states that Vasodilan is "possibly effective" for the symptomatic relief of vascular disorders claimed by the manufacturer.

The American Medical Association takes an even more critical view. In its publication, *AMA Drug Evaluations*, the AMA states that Vasodilan (isoxuprine) "increases muscle blood flow in normal individuals, but does not significantly affect blood flow to the skin. It does not improve calf muscle blood flow in patients with occlusive vascular disorders and is ineffective in relieving intermittent claudication. There is also no convincing evidence that isoxuprine [Vasodilan] is useful in vasospastic disorders, cerebrovascular disease, or other conditions for which it has been promoted."

Are there any special precautions?

Vasodilan should not be used soon after any surgical operation. The drug should be used with extreme caution (if at all) during pregnancy.

Vibramycin®

Generic name
Doxycycline

Class of drug
Broad-spectrum antibiotic

In what form is the drug available?
Capsules, syrup, and oral suspension (to be taken by mouth)

Why is the drug prescribed?
It is used mainly to treat a wide variety of microbial infections, including those caused by certain species of bacteria and rickettsiae (microorganisms intermediate in size between bacteria and viruses).

What are some possible side effects?
The most frequently encountered side effects include nausea, vomiting, and diarrhea. Some patients taking Vibramycin may occasionally have what is known as a photosensitivity reaction when exposed to strong sunlight. This can result in various types of skin eruptions and rashes, which are usually reversible once use of the drug has been discontinued.

The use of Vibramycin by children under the age of eight can cause permanent discoloration of their teeth. It can also cause discoloration of teeth in a fetus if the mother takes Vibramycin during the last half of pregnancy when the teeth are developing.

What should you know about the drug?

Vibramycin is a synthetic derivative of oxytetracycline, which is classed among the tetracycline group of drugs. Unlike most other tetracyclines, the therapeutic effects of Vibramycin are not significantly impaired if the drug is taken with meals or dairy products.

Are there any special precautions?

Vibramycin should *not* be used during pregnancy or during the nursing period.

Consult your physician before taking any other drugs at the same time as Vibramycin.

Vioform®-Hydrocortisone

Generic name

This product contains a combination of iodochlorhydroxyquin and hydrocortisone.

Class of drug

Topical corticosteroid, antibacterial, and antifungal agent

In what form is the drug available?

Cream, ointment, and lotion

Why is the drug prescribed?

It is used to treat various types of skin inflammation, including eczema, athlete's foot, and other fungal infections.

What are some possible side effects?

The most frequently encountered side effects are itching, burning sensations, irritation, skin rashes, and dry skin. The skin condition being treated may be made worse if the patient is sensitive (experiences an allergic reaction) to either of the ingredients of Vioform-Hydrocortisone.

This drug should not be used to treat virus infections of the skin such as chicken pox or shingles, since it may spread the infection.

Vioform-Hydrocortisone should not be applied to large areas of the skin or left on the skin for prolonged periods. The drug may be absorbed through the skin and cause various toxic (poisonous) reactions.

What should you know about the drug?

Prolonged use of Vioform-Hydrocortisone may result in the overgrowth of various species of microorganisms both bacterial and fungal. The National Science Foundation, National Research Council, and the FDA all report that the drug is only "possibly effective." Additional clinical research is presently being carried out.

Are there any special precautions?

If local skin irritation is noted during the use of Vioform-Hydrocortisone, discontinue its use and consult your physician at once.

Zyloprim®

Generic name
Allopurinol

Class of drug
Antihyperuricemic (antigout) agent

In what form is the drug available?
Tablets

Why is the drug prescribed?

It is used in the treatment of patients with chronic gout (gouty arthritis), a disorder of the body's metabolism. Gout causes an excruciatingly painful inflammation of one or more joints, typically the joint of the big toe. This results from the presence in the body fluids of an excess amount of uric acid (a waste product of metabolism which is normally flushed out of the body in the urine). When the concentration of uric acid reaches a certain level, crystals of uric acid form and are deposited in and around movable joints. This leads to inflammation of the affected joint.

Zyloprim acts by inhibiting the formation of excessive amounts of uric acid in the body. The drug is also used in other conditions where blood levels of uric acid are abnormally high (hyperuricemia) and unrelated to clinical evidence of gout, to prevent the formation of uric acid stones in the kidneys.

What are some possible side effects?

The most frequently encountered side effects are skin rashes and itching (pruritus). The incidence of skin rashes is unusually high in patients who are taking the antibiotic ampicillin at the same time as Zyloprim.

Some patients taking Zyloprim may experience nausea, vomiting, diarrhea, and intermittent abdominal pain. Other side effects are extremely rare.

What should you know about the drug?

Some experts believe that high levels of uric acid are best removed from the body by drugs known as uricosurics. These act by helping the kidneys to flush out uric acid in the urine. This is in contrast to the action of Zyloprim, which inhibits the excess formation of uric acid. However, uricosuric drugs cannot be used in patients with kidney damage.

Are there any special precautions?

Discontinue the use of Zyloprim at the first sign of any skin rash, and consult your physician.

Zyloprim should be used with caution (if at all) during pregnancy and during the nursing period. Take Zyloprim exactly as prescribed by your physician.

Table of drugs listed by type

Analgesics (pain relievers)

Darvocet-N 100
Darvon
Darvon Compound-65
Empirin Compound with Codeine
Equagesic
Fiorinal
Fiorinal with Codeine
Norgesic
Percodan
Phenaphen with Codeine
Pyridium
Synalgos-DC
Talwin
Tylenol with Codeine

Anorectics (appetite suppressants)

Ionamin
Tenuate

Antibacterials (antibiotics, sulfa drugs)

amoxicillin
ampicillin
Azo Gantrisin
Bactrim
Cortisporin Otic
erythromycin
Gantanol
Gantrisin
Keflex
Macrodantin
penicillin G
penicillin VK
tetracycline
Vibramycin

Anticoagulant (blood-clotting disorders)

Coumadin

Anticonvulsant (convulsions, epilepsy)

Dilantin

Antidiarrheal

Lomotil

Antiemetic (nausea & vomiting)

Tigan

Antifungals/antiparasitics

Flagyl
Kwell
Monistat
Mycolog
Mycostatin Vaginal Tablets
Vioform-Hydrocortisone

Antihistamines & decongestants

Actifed
Antivert
Benadryl
Bendectin
Chlor-Trimeton
Dimetane Expectorant
Dimetapp
Drixoral
Naldecon
Ornade
Periactin
Phenergan Expectorant
Phenergan VC Expectorant
Teldrin

Antihyperuricemic (gout)

Zyloprim

Anti-inflammatory drugs

Butazolidin Alka
Cordran
Indocin
Kenalog
Lidex
Medrol Tablets
Motrin
Nalfon
Naprosyn
prednisone
Synalar
Tandearil
Tolectin
Valisone

Antispasmodics (digestive tract)

Bentyl with
  Phenobarbital
Combid
Donnatal
Librax
Pro-Banthine

Antitussives (cough suppressants)

Actifed-C Expectorant
Ambenyl Expectorant
Phenergan Expectorant
  with Codeine
Phenergan VC
  Expectorant with
  Codeine
Tuss-Ornade

Bronchodilators/ antiasthmatics (breathing disorders)

Marax
Quibron

Dietary supplements

Poly-Vi-Flor
Slow-K

Gastric acid inhibitor

Tagamet

Heart & blood vessels

(high blood pressure,
tissue swelling, abnor-
mal heart rhythms, an-
gina pectoris, narrowed
blood vessels)

Aldactazide
Aldactone
Aldomet
Aldoril
Apresoline Hydrochloride
Catapres
Cyclospasmol
digoxin
Diupres
Diuril
Dyazide
Enduron
hydrochlorothiazide
Hydropres
Hygroton
Inderal
Isordil
Lasix
nitrogylcerin
Pavabid
Persantine
Pronestyl
quinidine sulfate
Regroton
Salutensin
Ser-Ap-Es
Vasodilan

Hormone therapy

Premarin
Proloid
Provera
Synthroid
thyroid

**Mental confusion &
 antisocial behavior
(elderly patients)**

Hydergine

Muscle relaxant

Parafon Forte

**Ophthalmic drugs
(eyes)**

Isopto-Carpine
Neosporin

Oral contraceptives

Demulen
Lo/Ovral
Norinyl
Norlestrin-21
Ortho-Novum
Ovral
Ovulen

**Oral hypoglycemics
(diabetes)**

Diabinese
Orinase
Tolinase

Sedatives & hypnotics

Butisol Sodium
Dalmane
Doriden
phenobarbital

**Serum lipid
(cholesterol)**

Atromid-S

Stimulant

Ritalin

**Tranquilizers &
antidepressants**

Atarax
Compazine
Elavil
Librium
Mellaril
meprobamate
Serax
Sinequan
Stelazine
Thorazine
Tofranil
Tranxene
Triavil
Valium

Index

183